The Strength Training Anatomy Workout

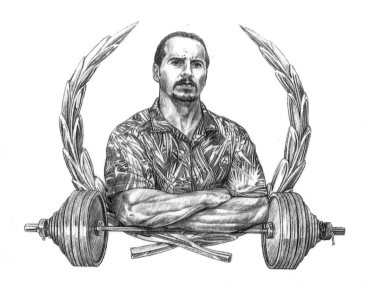

FRÉDÉRIC DELAVIER • MICHAEL GUNDILL

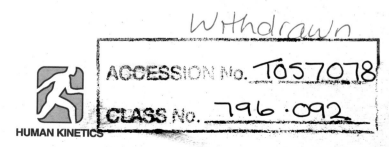

HUMAN KINETICS

CONTENTS

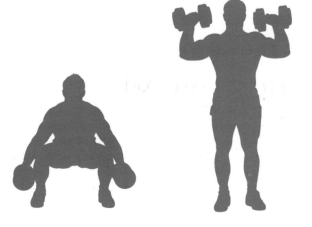

INTRODUCTION
Advantages of Working Out at Home

There are two major advantages to working out at home. First, there are practical aspects, and then there is the question of effectiveness. For these two reasons, one of the authors, Michael Gundill, chose to work out entirely at home, and the other author, Frédéric Delavier, did three-quarters of his workouts at home and the rest at a gym.

Practical Aspects of Exercising at Home

1 It can be difficult to find a good gym.

Unfortunately, there are very few good gyms for weight training. Many gyms invest in cardio and group classes rather than in weight training, and in many gyms, serious weight trainers are not welcome.

2 You save time and money.

Going to the gym can be tedious. You have to get dressed, drive to the gym, and change into your workout clothes. Then, after working out, you have to do it all again in the opposite order. All of this can take more time than the actual workout. Add to this the fact that membership costs are more and more expensive because of the amount of activities offered. But why pay for group classes, a pool, or something else when you only want to spend two to four hours a week lifting weights?

3 You have the freedom to exercise when you want to.

At a gym, you can exercise only when the gym is open, and you can be limited by crowds. Working out at home gives you flexibility. You can work out in the morning, in the evening, or on alternate mornings and evenings to make the best use of your time.

4 No age limit exists.

Many gyms do not allow people under the age of 16 to use their facilities. This does not mean that people cannot start lifting weights before the age of 16. Weight training will not stunt your growth! On the contrary: The earlier you start, the greater the benefits. In this case, the only solution is to work out at home.

Why Working Out at Home Is the Right Choice

1 First and foremost: You get results.
Weight training is more than a hobby. You must practice it seriously and not take it lightly. You are training to achieve results, not to pass the time. Unfortunately, most gyms do not want this kind of person as a member. Gyms emphasize the fun aspects of exercising and do not focus on effectiveness. This is why gyms often choose equipment that looks nice over equipment that works well.

2 You need a place that fits your program.
Gyms certainly have a more social quality than your home can offer, but being social does not make your workout effective. Often, the opposite is true. Many gym members are not really there to work out. They go there to pass some time and to meet people. Sometimes gym patrons think it is strange to see people who are seriously working out.

3 You avoid the equipment trap.
In many gyms, the equipment choices were made based on cost rather than effectiveness. As a result, you will find equipment that is not effective and does not work well with human anatomy. This equipment is dangerous for muscles and joints.

4 You have better concentration.
At home, no one will disturb you while you are exercising in order to discuss the weather or to tell you that you are not exercising the right way. You will be able to remain focused and have a faster, more productive workout.

5 It is the best way to achieve the workout you planned.
In a gym, your resting time is largely determined by other gym members. Your choice of exercises or equipment depends on what is available when you are working out. All of this rarely fits with the program you have set to meet your objectives. Circuit training, which is indispensable for athletes' weight training, is next to impossible in a gym. Working out at home grants you this freedom.

6 You eliminate ego.
In front of other people, so as not to seem silly, people might perform their repetitions haphazardly with the goal of lifting as much as possible. Ultimately, this will mean slower progress and a greater risk of injury. At home, there is no one to impress. You can focus on effective work and not worry about what other people think.

7 You already have advice from a good coach.
Between them, the authors of this book have more than 50 years of experience in fitness training. This is clearly more experience than that of most people you will meet at a gym who want to give you advice.

Develop Your Strength Training Program

At first, developing a personalized workout program might seem like a tedious chore. In fact, it is rather easy if you start with good goals and go in stages. This is the slow progression that we describe.

Equipment

For equipment, this book sets two conditions:

1. The equipment is inexpensive or free.
2. The space required for exercise is minimal.

It is possible to exercise without any equipment, but basic tools will increase the number of exercises you can do as well as their effectiveness. Ideally, you should have the following:

> A pair of dumbbells
> A pull-up bar
> Elastic bands

You will use your bed, a door frame, and a chair to perform these exercises.

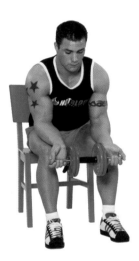

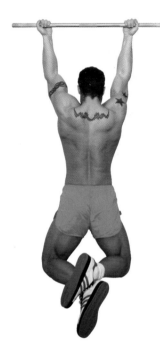

▍Dumbbells

Adjustable dumbbells are available in any sporting goods store. A 20-pound (approximately 10 kg) kit costs around $20. Ideally, you should have two kits. Then, as you become stronger, you can purchase additional weights as you need them.

The point in using dumbbells is to increase the difficulty of the exercises so that you continue to make progress. If you always do exercise with the same weight (your body weight, for example), even if you increase the number of repetitions and sets, you will rapidly reach a plateau. In weight training, everything is based on the principle of overload. Using dumbbells is the best way to reach this overload.

Instead of dumbbells, you can use bottles filled with water (the amount of water depends on the resistance that you want). Large bottles with handles (similar to milk jugs) are easier to use.

▍Pull-Up Bar

This is a moveable bar that you attach above the door-frame or between two walls in a hallway. After use, it can be stored away so it does not take up space. This bar is used in working the back, but it is not required.

There are short bars (less than 4 feet, or about a meter) and longer bars (up to 4 feet). If you have the room, choose longer bars. They will give you greater diversity in the exercises you can do.

▍Elastic Bands

Elastic bands or tubes are available in any sporting goods store. Some hardware stores also sell them.

The advantage of elastic bands is that they provide significant resistance but do not weigh anything. Bands are easy to transport and store at home. Ideally, you

Two ways to attach an elastic band

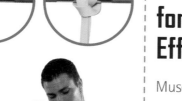

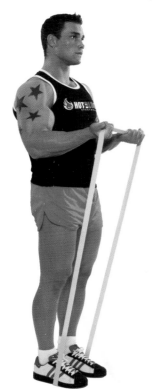

Diversify Resistance for Maximum Effectiveness

Muscular progression is even more rapid when you use various kinds of resistance.

For this reason, we recommend using not just one but five types of resistance:

1. Body-weight training
2. Additional resistance
3. Elastic resistance
4. Plyometric resistance
5. Stretching

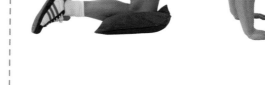

should have bands in several diameters or thicknesses so that you can easily vary the resistance.

The resistance provided by elastic bands is very different than that provided by the body or by a weight. The more you pull on a band, the greater the resistance. However, if you lift a 20-pound dumbbell, it will always weigh 20 pounds whether you are at the beginning, middle, or end of a movement.

Still, it would not be wise to choose one type of resistance over another. Both dumbbells and bands have their advantages and disadvantages in terms of resistance. One is not better than the other. The best method is to combine the two as often as possible. Combining them allows you to enjoy all the benefits while eliminating the drawbacks to both. This synergy provides a kind of resistance that is superior to all others.

We develop this concept further throughout this book.

▌Body-Weight Training

This is the basis for weight training. The advantages are that it does not require any equipment and all of the muscles in the body can be worked. Unfortunately, when body-weight training reaches a certain point in terms of strength and endurance, it quickly reaches its limits.

As in all disciplines, in order to improve, you must increase the difficulty. One of the ways to do this is to increase the number of repetitions. But if you go beyond 25 repetitions in body-weight training, you move from strength training to endurance training. For building size and strength in the muscles, increasing repetitions is not as effective as increasing weight.

9

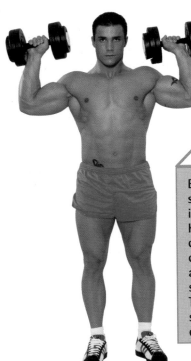

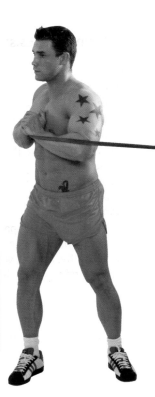

**INVOLUNTARY STRENGTH:
A PROGRESSIVE DEPOSIT!**

Even if you wanted to, you could not use all the strength in your muscles. Their total strength is enormous. You often realize this when you have a muscle cramp because it causes a muscle contraction that is much stronger than any you could voluntarily generate. The total strength of a muscle is the sum of its maximum voluntary strength plus its absolute involuntary strength. The difference between maximum voluntary strength and absolute involuntary strength is called the strength deficit.

▌Additional Resistance

To increase the difficulty of an exercise and to force the muscle to grow, you must push it. The easiest way to do this is by using dumbbells. Dumbbells allow you to vary the resistance gradually. It is possible to add just one pound (about .5 kg) at a time or more if you have the strength. This progressive addition of weight is the opposite of that provided by body weight, which does not vary. Many people cannot do pull-ups or push-ups. With dumbbells, this is never an issue since you can select any weight you like.

Dumbbells are an extension of body-weight training, but they are less restrictive for people who are new to weight training and who have not yet gained enough strength for body-weight training. With dumbbells, stronger athletes can go beyond using only their body weight by increasing the weight voluntarily and gradually.

▌Elastic Resistance

We have already explained that the nature of elastic resistance is very different than that provided by dumbbells or your body weight. To vary the resistance of elastic bands, you have two choices:

1. Play with the tension—the more you stretch a band, the more resistance you encounter.
2. Use different kinds of bands and therefore different strengths.

Selecting resistance in this way is less precise than when using dumbbells, but it allows more variation than that provided by your body weight. Training with dumbbells or body weight means the muscle has to rely on voluntary strength to increase the weight. With a band, the role of absolute involuntary strength is much greater. In this way, the band represents a transition between traditional resistance and plyometrics. In effect, when you pull on a band, the final movement quickly brings you back to the starting position. This kind of training is similar to the quick movements of plyometrics. For a more in-depth explanation of this, see the section titled Negatives on page 46. To progress quickly, you must both increase the total strength of the muscle and infringe as much as possible on absolute involuntary strength (in other words, reduce the strength deficit). Plyometric training as well as resistance provided by bands will allow you to do just that.

Plyometric Resistance

Plyometric resistance (also called the stretch-shortening cycle) gives muscles elastic and rebound properties. This resistance comes into play when you force your muscles to abruptly stop a movement and then go in the opposite direction. A typical example of plyometric effort is to jump off a short box, land while absorbing the shock, and use it to jump as high and as fast as possible. Running uses this phenomenon of plyometric rebounding as well. This is why, when you train using plyometrics, you end up running faster and jumping higher. The muscle becomes more explosive.

Plyometric work is particularly important for athletes who need muscle reactivity. By causing a small, quick stretch of the muscle, you cause a protective reflex: the myotatic reflex. It greatly mobilizes absolute involuntary strength. This can be seen in elite sprinters. Watch them hop in place before the start of a race. With little momentum, they can jump very high and extremely fast. This plyometric effort before the start prepares the muscles to use all their explosiveness in the race.

Plyometrics brings together the strength gained through weight training and the increase in performance on the field. An athlete can become stronger through weight training, but when you ask him, for example, to throw a small ball, he cannot throw it very far because it is difficult for him to transform his strength into explosiveness; his muscles are not accustomed to that type of movement. When he quickly brings his arm back to throw the ball, the interaction between the involuntary strength generated and the voluntary muscle contraction is often not a direct carryover. Plyometrics can help you transform your strength into explosiveness.

Plyometrics primarily involves the thighs as well as the upper-body muscles you might use to push an opponent away or to pitch a baseball.

The golden rule in plyometrics is to limit contact with the floor. If contact lasts too long, a good part of the myotatic reflex is lost. The goal of plyometrics is to accelerate maximum voluntary muscle growth so that it adds itself as rapidly as possible to the involuntary strength (mobilized by abrupt stretching). Letting the shockwave from contact with the floor dissipate for too long (even milliseconds too long) means the interaction does not happen in the optimal time frame. Involuntary strength fades before enough voluntary strength has even been mobilized. In the example of the athlete throwing a ball, the time available to make the throw is extremely short. Poor interaction between the two kinds of strength results in a bad throw because the athlete was not able to gather all of his strength in that very brief period.

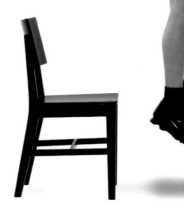

Measuring fatigue during plyometric exercise is very different from measuring it during classic exercise. You must stop plyometric exercise when the time of contact with the floor becomes too long. In this case, the explosiveness will no longer be worked enough and poor habits (muscle slowness) will begin. As soon as the time of contact with the floor increases and you have less explosiveness, the set should be interrupted. This rule makes the determination of how much to do in plyometrics fairly easy. Three or four sets of one to three plyometric exercises are generally more than sufficient.

For this reason, you should not do too many plyometric exercises, because they can become counterproductive. When the thigh muscles are really warmed up, you can begin with a few plyometric exercises, a little like the sprinters who wake up their nervous systems by doing jumps before a race. However, we do not advise you to end a very tiring thigh workout with plyometrics. In that case, the interaction between involuntary strength and voluntary strength could be slowed because of fatigue.

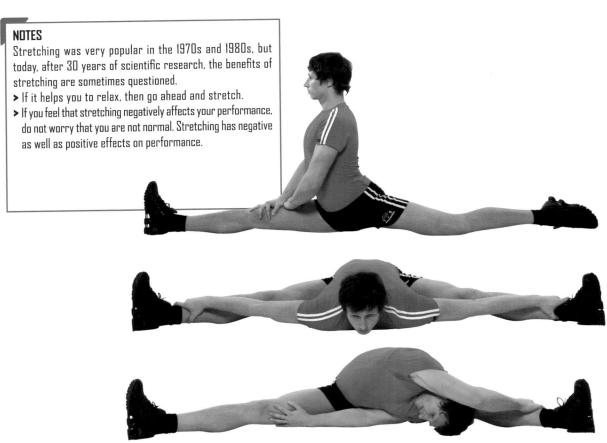

▌Stretching

Stretching plays on the strength of the muscle's passive resistance. Constant strength training can reduce the range of motion by tightening muscles. A certain amount of tightness is necessary, especially in strength sports, but too much tension and a restricted range of motion can result in injuries. However, flexibility is not an end in itself. Flexibility is impressive, but beyond a certain point, too much flexibility will work against performance.

> **We believe that stretching a muscle can either increase or inhibit performance, so you must be very careful to stretch properly.**

You must find a good compromise between muscle tightness and flexibility. This compromise was defined by the Soviet bodybuilding masters: To prevent injuries, muscles must remain flexible enough to have a slightly larger range of motion than is needed in your sport, but not so much that you lose strength.

You need to stretch muscles in the following four instances:

1 During warm-up

If you stretch a rubber band for a few seconds, it will start to heat up. In the same way, stretching warms up muscles and tendons. But if you pull the rubber band too far, it will stretch out and lose its strength. It could even snap. Muscles are very similar. You must be gentle in stretching during the warm-up. In fact, medical research shows that warm-ups with sustained stretching are generally associated with reduced performance. Losing even a little bit of its reactivity will cause a muscle to be suddenly less explosive, because the stretch-shortening cycle is slower. This reduced performance lasts only a few hours, but it is enough to hinder a workout. So be careful not to overdo it when you stretch during a warm-up.

2 Between sets

During training, stretching can have two consequences:

1. In the best case, stretching allows you to rapidly regain muscle strength, which helps reduce the resting time between sets.
2. In the worst case, stretching can accentuate a loss of strength.

The explanations for both of these extremes are not as surprising as they might seem. They depend to a large degree on the amount of muscle fatigue achieved during the exercise. It could even be that stretching is beneficial between the first few sets and then counterproductive between the following sets. The opposite could also be true.

The advantage of stretching is that you feel its benefits or drawbacks right after the stretch. So you should not be too strict about stretching between sets. Even if some people praise the virtues of stretching, the benefits do not apply in every case and for every person all of the time.

3 After working out

This is the best time to stretch because even if there is a temporary reduction in performance, it will not be an issue. Ideally, you should stretch the muscles you have just worked because they are really warm. But keep in mind the rule we have explained: Being too flexible can harm your performance in the long run. Simply maintain a good range of motion so you can prevent injuries.

4 Between workouts

Stretching can be used to speed recovery between two workouts. The problem with this strategy is that you start with cold muscles, which can be dangerous. However, contrary to popular belief, stretching between workouts will not always help muscle recovery.

How to Stretch

Two main stretching techniques exist:

1 Static stretching

This involves simply holding the stretch for a certain amount of time (generally 10 seconds to 1 minute). The stretch can be very light or very strong, depending on your goal.

ADVANTAGES

If practiced with control and in a progressive manner, it is unlikely to cause injury.

- -

This type of stretching is more likely to reduce performance when it is done before a workout.

DISADVANTAGES

2 Ballistic stretching

This involves pulling on the muscles using small, abrupt movements that are repeated for 10 to 20 seconds. This kind of stretching resembles plyometrics because it involves the stretch-shortening cycle and causes a myotatic reflex contraction. The goal of these small movements is to force the muscles to stretch more than they naturally would.

ADVANTAGES

This type of stretching is less likely to reduce performance when it is done before a workout if you do not tear a muscle.

- -

You must be extremely careful with this type of stretching because it is more likely to cause an injury.

DISADVANTAGES

In general, you should do one to three sets of stretches per muscle group.

Conclusion

By using these five types of resistance (body weight, additional resistance, elastic resistance, plyometric resistance, and stretching), you will make the best use of all the types of strength that muscles can generate. The greater the range of your strengths, the faster you will progress.

How a Muscle Gains Strength

The bigger a muscle is, the stronger it will be. However, you probably know of someone who is very strong but does not have large muscles. How can this paradox be explained? Muscle size is only one of the factors that determine muscle strength. The power of a muscle's contraction depends on the following five things:

1. Number of Motor Neurons Used

A strong person is someone who has the ability to use the maximum amount of his muscle fibers at a given moment. The use of these muscle fibers is carried out by the central nervous system.

Everything starts at the cerebral level: The command given to contract muscles goes through the nerves in the spinal cord. Motor neurons then carry the command to the muscle fibers. Each motor neuron controls the contraction of a specific group of fibers. The more motor neurons that are activated, the greater the quantity of muscle fibers that will contract. This is why training should be done with heavy weights. The heavier the weight you lift, the more motor nerves you will be able to use simultaneously.

2. Strength of the Impulse Sent by Each Motor Neuron

Motor neurons can send electrical impulses to muscles with varying frequency. If the frequency is low, the muscle contracts sluggishly. However, motor neurons can send a flurry of intense impulses that act powerfully on muscle fibers. The intensity of your training develops your capacity to do the most repetitions possible with a heavy weight. Doing plyometrics also plays an important part in increasing the power of nerve impulses.

3. Size of the Muscle

There is a strict correlation between the size of muscle fibers and the strength they are capable of developing. The stronger a section of muscle fibers that is linked to a motor neuron, the more force will be generated by a nerve impulse. You can develop muscle mass by performing weight training exercises with a weight that is around 80 percent of your maximum strength.

4. Intramuscular Coordination

In a sedentary person, when motor neurons discharge their electrical impulses, they do so in a disorderly fashion. The muscle fibers contract in a random, and therefore inefficient, way. Through training, these discharges become synchronized. The fibers begin contracting in a coordinated manner. Muscles become more efficient. You can achieve this by doing weight training exercises with a weight that is close to your repetition maximum.

5. Intermuscular Coordination

It is rare that you have to contract only one muscle at a time. Generally, a whole group of muscles is activated to produce a movement. When resistance becomes greater, the muscles of inexperienced athletes have a hard time working together in an efficient manner. You can see this when such athletes do pull-ups. They lean to one side more than the other. They cannot pull themselves up in a linear fashion and without jerky movements. The body shifts from front to back.

Through training, the quality of movement improves, simply because the arms will have learned to work together with the back muscles, and the muscles on the right side will be in synch with the muscles on the left side.

This gain in efficiency translates to an increase in strength. It is the same in all areas of fitness when you have to learn a new move. It is the volume of work, and therefore the repetition of a movement or an exercise, that improves intermuscular coordination.

Through regular weight training, an athlete's muscles become accustomed to working together. This advanced work means that an athlete can learn new movements more quickly if he has already been weight training for months.

In summary, among the elements we have described, the size of a muscle is just one of five factors of strength. To increase power and strength, your weight training program must also improve the four factors that are part of the central nervous system.

Practical Consequences

You should glean several practical consequences from these physiological facts:

1 Rapid gains in strength that occur when you start weight training are not because of enlargement of the fibers. They are best explained by improvements in inter- and intramuscular coordination.

2 Therefore, just because you gain strength, at least in the beginning, it does not mean that your weight training program is well structured and that it will continue to help you progress quickly. Someone who is training well can gain strength if only because he is learning to execute movements better.

3 A beginner's gain in strength can be misleading. However, it is still better to gain strength than to lose it. If that happened, it would mean everything was going wrong.

4 You will notice that you are stronger on certain days. The size of your muscles has not changed, so the efficiency of the central nervous system is the explanation for these fluctuations in muscle power. When the central nervous system is well rested, it will demonstrate its efficiency and you will be strong. If the central nervous system has not fully recovered and is tired, then any weight you lift will seem heavier than it actually is.

5 These fluctuations in the central nervous system can create surprises, both good and bad. Before starting a certain training session, you might feel ready to tackle anything, when in fact you are not going to break any of your records. However, there will be days when you feel tired but will be surprised by your own strength because your central nervous system is well rested.

6 A well-rested central nervous system and well-rested muscles do not always coincide. The fact that recovery differs for each makes the task of planning your training that much more difficult.

Mechanisms of Muscle Enlargement

The tension your muscles are subjected to regulates their size.

In the absence of weight, muscle mass melts away. This is why astronauts' muscles atrophy rapidly in space. Weight training produces the opposite effect. By subjecting muscles to significant tension, they have to reinforce themselves and grow larger.

Muscle enlargement basically happens through the addition of the contractile elements actin and myosin (muscle filaments in charge of contracting muscles). The body also has the ability to increase the number of muscle fibers through proliferation of the stem cells they contain. These stem cells (also called satellite cells) will transform themselves into muscle cells in reaction to the tension generated by regular training.

However, this growth process is not nearly as simple as it sounds. One training session is not going to make your muscles bigger. The very first result of a training session is damage to the muscle fibers. This is why you lose strength and feel sore after any physical effort. Weight training is a kind of destruction (or catabolism) of muscles. This is why you must not train excessively (see the special section titled Overtraining on page 16).

Fortunately, your body will react to this abuse. It will try to repair the damaged parts of the muscle. All the magic of the human body involves following a repair with reinforcement (or overcompensation) of the muscle structure. Thus, instead of just fixing itself, your body will synthesize new actin and myosin filaments. Over time, these excess filaments lead to an increase in muscle mass. Thanks to these additions, your muscles will be stronger and ready to resist the catabolic effect of weight training sessions.

20 Steps to Developing Your Program

You now have all the basic theory required for developing your program. Creating your program will take 20 steps, which we describe in detail. When you have finished this section, you will have answered all your questions about developing your training program. You will also discover why you must constantly change your program as a function of your muscle growth.

1. How many times per week should you train?

To answer this first question, your schedule will be a determining factor. Unfortunately, this is not always optimal. But know that if you can train only once a week, this is still better than zero times a week. You will still make progress. For athletes who are already training intensely for their sports, one weight training session per week will suffice. However, it seems that two weight training sessions per week are a good minimum. For people who do not do any other activities other than weight training, the ideal would probably be three times a week. We still recommend that you not do more than four training sessions per week. Keep in mind that overtraining is more damaging to your progress than undertraining. Only excellent athletes will benefit from more than four sessions per week.

! When you start weight training, you are generally full of enthusiasm and energy. You feel like working out every day so you can make a lot of progress. This much enthusiasm at the beginning could turn into disillusionment as well as fatigue (overtraining), and then you could lose motivation. Athletes who know how to ration their efforts will get the most benefit from weight training. The results will not happen instantly, so you must be patient.

Evolution

Ideally, you should start with two weekly sessions for a month or two before moving to three sessions when you feel ready. At first, do not work out more than three times per week. After three to six months of regular training, a four-day program could be planned.

2. Which days should you train?

Ideally, you should alternate one day of training with one day of rest. Here again, this might not work well with your schedule. In that case, you have to find a balance between the ideal and what is possible for you. Here are options with various programs:

> **One workout per week.** You can choose any day you like.

> **Two workouts per week.** Weight training sessions should be spaced out as far as possible (for example, Monday and Thursday or Tuesday and Friday). In any case, give yourself at least one day of rest between two workouts. The exception is if you are able to work out only on the weekends. Working out two consecutive days is not ideal, but you will have the rest of the week to recover.

> **Three workouts per week.** The best plan would be to alternate a day of training with a day of rest. For example, train on Monday, Wednesday, and Friday. This way your whole weekend is free. It is still possible to do two days of training consecutively (on the weekend, for example) and do the third training on Wednesday. But you should avoid this as much as possible. The worst program would have you training three days in a row. The only way to justify this is if your schedule absolutely requires it.

> **Four workouts per week.** In this schedule, you have the fewest number of rest days, and therefore you will have to work out two days in a row. If you are doing four workouts per week, this means you are working the upper body once and the legs once (see the following page). So you should ensure that the upper-body workout is followed by the leg workout. Your schedule will be Monday, Wednesday, Friday, and Sunday, or Tuesday, Thursday, Saturday, and Monday.

If your schedule is very flexible, you could do your training sessions over eight days instead of seven. Thus, one day of training will always be followed by one day of rest. Recovery will be optimized because of the slightly longer training intervals. The only inconvenience is that your training days will change from week to week on this program.

3. How many times per week should you work each muscle?

For athletes who are accustomed to serious weight training, one weekly session could be enough. This means working each muscle only once per week. But it would be difficult to increase this interval, at least at first. You could increase the frequency of your workouts when you have more free time.

For those who want to make quick progress in volume and strength, the best thing to do is to work each muscle group two or three times per week.

> **NOTE**
> There is a fundamental difference between bodybuilding for muscle mass and training to increase athletic performance. In the latter case, all the muscles should be worked on the same day, because in most sports, muscles work together and not individually. The artificial distinction between different muscle groups applies especially to those who want larger muscles for aesthetic reasons.

Evolution

Start by working all of your muscles during each of your two weekly training sessions. After two to three weeks at this pace, if you feel ready, you can increase to three weekly sessions in which you will work all muscle groups each time. To ensure a smooth transition, you could alternate one week with two workouts and one week with three workouts, and so on, until you feel comfortable with three sessions per week. However, working each muscle three times per week might be too much, especially if you have other training specifically for your sport.

Later, you will reach a point where it will no longer be possible to work all muscle groups in a single session. This is when you will need to move to a different schedule. That schedule can include three or four training days.

Three-Day Schedule

This schedule allows you to track your priorities and your weak points.

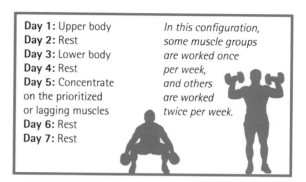

Day 1: Upper body
Day 2: Rest
Day 3: Lower body
Day 4: Rest
Day 5: Concentrate on the prioritized or lagging muscles
Day 6: Rest
Day 7: Rest

In this configuration, some muscle groups are worked once per week, and others are worked twice per week.

Four-Day Schedule

This schedule allows you to work the upper and lower body twice a week. To overcome the greater intensity of training on a four-day schedule, the training frequency for each muscle is limited to twice per week instead of three times per week.

If your program runs over two weeks instead of one, each group will be worked three times in 14 days. The muscles will then have three or four days to recover between workouts. We do not advise that you work all muscles four times a week. This frequency will not allow enough time for the muscles to fully recover because they will have only one or two days between each workout.

This is an example of a program with equal work between upper-body and lower-body muscles:

Day 1: Upper body
Day 2: Rest
Day 3: Lower body
Day 4: Rest
Day 5: Upper body
Day 6: Lower body
Day 7: Rest

This is an example of a program with more upper-body work:

Day 1: Upper body
Day 2: Rest
Day 3: Upper body
Day 4: Rest
Day 5: Upper body
Day 6: Lower body
Day 7: Rest

Knowing how many times a week to work a muscle involves deciding how many rest days to allow between workouts. Muscle grows only during the rest phase between workouts and not during the workout itself. It is just as important to know how to rest as it is to know how to train. The problem is that all of the muscles do not necessarily recover at the same rate. Certain muscles recover more quickly than others. You will quickly realize this because certain muscle groups will grow stronger than others. It would be wise to allow more resting time for the muscles that are weaker, because this is a sign that they need more rest.

4. Should you exercise once or twice per day?

Champion athletes are not the only ones who exercise more than once a day. And they are not necessarily preparing for a competition, either! But for others, it is better to exercise only once a day and not every single day.

If you can work out only once a week because of your schedule, you might eventually want to divide that training workout in two (not at first, of course, but after a few weeks of training). Dividing the session in two will allow you to continue to make progress. This is, however, far from an ideal program.

5. What time of day should you work out?

Some people prefer to train in the morning and others in the afternoon or evening. In fact, strength varies depending on the time of day. Some people are stronger in the mornings and weaker in the afternoon. For others the opposite is true. These fluctuations due to the central nervous system are completely normal. It is rare to find athletes who have consistent strength throughout the day.

Ideally, you should train when your muscles are the strongest! The majority of athletes are strongest around 6 to 7 p.m. This works out well since many people exercise at that time.

Your workout time may be determined by your daily schedule and not by your body. Even if you are not training at the best time for your body, a simple rule is that you should always work out at the same time each day. Your muscles will get used to it, and this way they will perform their best at that time.

6. How many muscles should you work during a training session?

The body is made up of six muscle groups:

1. Arms (biceps, triceps, forearms)
2. Shoulders
3. Chest
4. Back
5. Abdomen
6. Legs (quadriceps, hamstrings, glutes, and calves).

Should you work each of the muscles during every workout or only do a few groups per training session?

The answer to this question will depend largely on the number of times you work out per week. When you begin with a program that includes one, two, or three workouts a week, it is best to work out the entire body on one day. Since each muscle is stimulated with just a few sets, the total volume of the training session is manageable. Over time, you will add sets for each muscle, and the volume of work will become too much for one workout. You will determine when it is too difficult to work all the muscles on the same day.

It will then become necessary to divide your program into several workouts. Dividing in this way is called doing a split. A split lowers the frequency with which each muscle is stimulated during any given week. In exchange, you can increase the intensity and the volume of work for each muscle since there will be fewer groups to work during each session. We advise you to do weight training regularly for two to three months before splitting your workouts.

A split is possible only when you are doing at least two weekly workouts. Instead of doing the six muscle groups in a single session, you will work four groups during one workout and the rest on another day.

Here is a split over two days:

SESSION 1	SESSION 2
Upper body (shoulders, chest, back, arms)	Lower body, abdomen

A split over three sessions could look like this:

SESSION 1	SESSION 2	SESSION 3
Upper body (shoulders, chest, back, arms)	Lower body, abdomen	Upper body (chest, back, shoulders, arms)

This split highlights the upper-body muscles to the detriment of the legs. It is suitable for athletes for whom the legs are not a priority.

A program based on four workouts per week is the most appropriate in order to develop a split that is balanced between the upper body and lower body.

SESSION 1	SESSION 3
Upper body (back, shoulders, chest, arms)	Upper body (chest, shoulders, back, arms)
SESSION 2	**SESSION 4**
Lower body (quadriceps, hamstrings, calves)	Lower body (hamstrings, quadriceps, calves)

If your legs are not a priority, the following split might work for you:

SESSION 1	SESSION 3
Chest, back	Chest, back, arms
SESSION 2	**SESSION 4**
Shoulders, arms	Shoulders, thighs

What you should understand here is the progressive logic that drives each evolution. Ideally, you should balance each workout as much as possible in terms of volume of work, duration, and intensity. From there, you can do any kind of split.

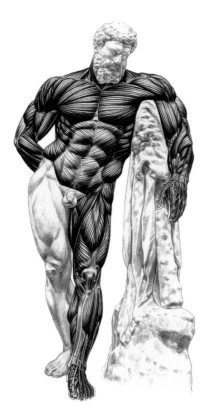
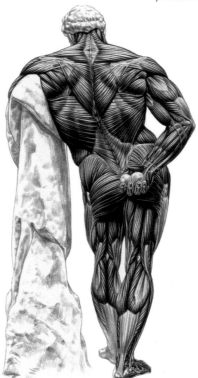
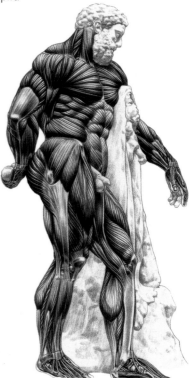

7. In what order should you work the muscles?

Statistically, there are many possible combinations for working the six major muscle groups, but they are not all good. We will explain how to reduce the number of combinations so that you can focus on the most effective combinations.

A good order for working the muscles depends on four things:
1. Simple rules to follow
2. The priority you have assigned to each muscle group
3. Your weak areas
4. The principle of rotation

1 The rules

There are a few rules that apply to most people who want bigger muscles:

> Do not work your arms before your chest, shoulders, or back. For these three groups, you will need all the strength in your arms. Your arm muscles must not be too tired when you begin working the torso muscles. The only exception would be for athletes who are concentrating on their arms and not the rest of the body.

> The same goes for the legs. Always work the calves last. When they are tired, they might begin to shake when you really push the thighs. This shaking not only will decrease your performance, but it could also be dangerous because you could fall.

> Even if you want a well-balanced body, it is better to work the upper body before the lower body. One reason you should not work the thighs first is their size. After you work your legs, you will be very tired, and then you still have to work the upper-body muscles. Unless legs are your priority, keep this rule in mind so that you do not adversely affect your upper-body workout.

> Do not work an upper-body muscle, then a lower-body muscle, and then go back to the upper body (for example, chest, quadriceps, shoulders, hamstrings, back). This type of workout has value for those who do specific sports, but not for people who want to increase muscle mass. As much as possible, work muscles that are close together (for example, chest, then shoulders, then back).

These rules do not apply to circuit training, which is based on an entirely different system than the maximum use of weaker muscles.

2 Your priorities

The second item that will determine the order in which you train your muscles is your priorities.

For people who want muscle mass, all muscles are not necessarily treated the same way. For example, many people give the upper body greater priority and let the lower body falter. This choice allows them to make quick aesthetic progress.

If you want chiseled abdominal muscles, you can begin each workout with abdominal work as a kind of warm-up. If those muscles are not a priority, you can work them at the end of a session. You can work the abdominal muscles more or less intensely depending on your energy level and how much time you have left to work out.

Athletes must create a hierarchy of importance for each muscle group depending on their sport. For example, for a shot-putter, the shoulders, triceps, quadriceps, and abdominal muscles are especially important.

For a soccer player, the priority will be the quadriceps rather than the upper body. For a swimmer, upper-body muscles are most important, but the quadriceps are not neglected.

Your priorities should be reflected in the structure of your training program. You must keep in mind that when you emphasize certain muscles, other muscles will be neglected a bit since you have a limited capacity for high-intensity training.

3 Your weak areas

You should always emphasize your weak areas. It is rare that all muscles progress at the same rate. If you want bigger muscles, and if your chest is more important than your shoulders, then you will train your shoulders before your chest.

Using our previous example, a shot-putter would normally begin his circuit with quadriceps, then work the shoulders, and finish with the triceps. But if what prevents him from throwing farther is a lack of strength in his arms, then the training order for these muscle groups could be reversed so that triceps are emphasized. Demonstrating flexibility, he could also start his first weekly training session with arms and his second weekly training session with quads. This is the principle of rotation.

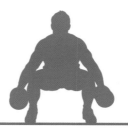

4 Principle of rotation

This principle will solve many of the problems encountered when you first begin working out. Rotation means constantly alternating the order of the muscle groups that you work first during each session. The advantage of rotation is that you avoid a routine that could quickly become tedious. Keeping your routine fresh will help you maintain a high level of motivation.

You can also plan a rotation concerning the muscles you want to emphasize temporarily. For example, during one month you concentrate on your chest and do not work your deltoids as hard so that you do not stress your shoulder joints. The next month, you do the opposite.

Sample Programs

Here are some examples of training programs for muscle groups that you can adapt to your needs. We provide them as a way to illustrate the number of possibilities that are available. See sections 1, 2, and 3 in part 3 of this book for more detailed programs.

Programming:

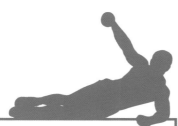

One Training Session per Week

More so than with other programs, the choice of which muscles to work first in each session is critical here. Indeed, as your training progresses, you will become more and more tired. You will then have less strength to work the muscle groups at the end of your session.

The main thing to keep in mind is your priorities. If you only want to build up your chest, then each session starts with your chest muscles. If you want to build up your chest and shoulders, then alternate sessions that begin with the shoulders and sessions that begin with the chest muscles.

If you are focusing on your arms, the program will be a bit more complex for the reasons just explained. In this case, start with the arms and choose isolation exercises that do not emphasize them too much, and then work the torso muscles.

Two Training Sessions per Week

The principle of rotation is easier to apply here. You will want to make the best use of the principle by beginning as many sessions as possible with different muscle groups. For the upper body, alternate between chest, back, and shoulders to start your workout. For the lower body, you can alternate between quadriceps and hamstrings. You could begin with glutes, but you may tire out your legs this way. Do this only if the glutes are your priority.

Three Training Sessions per Week

The strategy remains the same as for two training sessions per week. The advantage of having more workouts per week is that you have even more opportunities to rotate exercises.

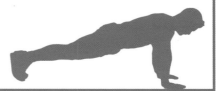

Four Training Sessions per Week

With this more advanced structure, the upper and lower split comes naturally. It is possible to work the upper body and lower body twice each, but you could also work the upper body three times and the lower body only once, depending on your priorities. In this more frequent training program, the rotation of muscle groups on the same day is not as important.

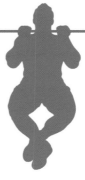

8. How many sets should you do for each muscle?

The amount of work for each muscle is determined by two criteria:

1. The number of sets per exercise
2. The number of exercises per muscle

   Your level will determine the approximate number of sets that you should perform.

> ### DEFINITION
> A **set** is the number of repetitions of the same movement until you reach fatigue. The number of sets done per muscle is an important factor for muscular development. If you do too many sets, you will overwork the muscle, which will prevent it from growing. If you do not do enough sets, the muscle will not be stimulated optimally so it can grow rapidly.

Beginners
For small muscles, do no more than two or three sets total. For large muscles, do no more than three or four sets.

After One Month of Training
For small muscles, do no more than four sets. For large muscles, do no more than five sets.

After Two Months of Training
For small muscles, do no more than five sets. For large muscles, do no more than six sets.

After Three Months of Training
For small muscles, do no more than six sets. For large muscles, do no more than seven sets.

After three months, you will be comfortable choosing your own number of sets based on your needs for each muscle as well as their capacity for recovery.

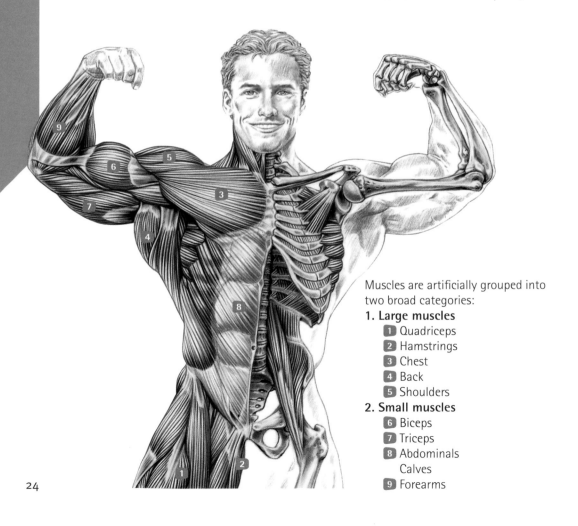

Muscles are artificially grouped into two broad categories:
1. **Large muscles**
   1. Quadriceps
   2. Hamstrings
   3. Chest
   4. Back
   5. Shoulders
2. **Small muscles**
   6. Biceps
   7. Triceps
   8. Abdominals
      Calves
   9. Forearms

! ● If you have no difficulty going beyond these limits, this means your muscle contraction intensity is not high enough. This intensity comes with time as you train. You may not necessarily be able to push your physical possibilities to the limit in a set from one day to the next. But you are not just doing easy sets until you reach a magic number, either. It is better to ask more of yourself in every set and end up doing fewer total sets.

Flexibility

The number of sets is the first adjustable variable in the volume of work for a given muscle. It is a more refined adjustment than the addition of exercises. At first, you must play around with adding sets rather than increase the number of exercises for a given muscle. As you become stronger and when you feel ready, add a set here and there.

The best thing is to let your muscles tell you how many sets you should do. The most obvious indicator is when you start to lose strength abnormally from one set to the next. An abrupt loss of strength indicates that you have perhaps done one set too many. You will know this when you do your next workout.

Obviously, the number of sets that you are able to do can fluctuate from one session to the next. On days when you are feeling great, you might be tempted to add sets. But on days when you are feeling tired, you can reduce the number of sets so that you do not wear yourself out.

You must also keep in mind what you did in the previous workout. If you increased your weight and your sets, you must also expect that your recovery time will be longer. This is why a really good workout is often followed by a poor workout. Because you asked more of your body, it has not had enough time to fully recover. So that the following workouts do not suffer, it is important to take one day of rest between two workouts.

CONTROVERSY SURROUNDING SINGLE OR MULTIPLE SETS

There is great controversy concerning the number of sets you should do for each muscle. Some say that one very intense set per exercise should suffice. This is true for certain athletes whose central nervous system has the capacity to give its maximum effort for one intense set. Afterward, they lose a lot of strength and cannot repeat the same effort. In this case, doing a second set of the exercise would be counterproductive. Very few people's central nervous systems have this characteristic. Scientific research estimates that about 70 percent of athletes do better with multiple sets. Only the remaining 30 percent have muscles that are better adapted for single sets.

Most athletes need to increase intensity gradually so they can give their maximum to the workout. With a single set per exercise, they feel frustrated because their muscles have not been able to fully express their power. They still have strength left over for another set. In this case, it would be counterproductive to do only one set per exercise. For those people, the best thing is to do several sets so the muscles can really work.

Multiple sets are also more appropriate for athletes than for nonathletes. Doing two or three sets per exercise means

- performing the first set on a fresh muscle,
- performing the second set on a muscle that is not really tired, and
- performing the third set on a tired muscle.

This is the type of work required of an athlete. It is rare to have a discipline that requires a single intense effort before the athlete is finished. Even for sprinters, there are elimination rounds before the final. So you must get in the habit of asking a lot of a muscle that has already been used. When training using only single sets, you will be great at elimination rounds, but you will crumble afterward because you will not be used to giving your all when your muscles are already tired from a previous intense effort.

9. How many exercises should you do for each muscle?

When you begin, you should choose a single exercise (one that is best suited for you—we explain how to choose it later on) for each muscle and for each workout. This rule applies when you are working all of your muscle groups during the same workout. You can increase the number of exercises when you begin splitting workouts.

You can add exercises later to accentuate the work of the large muscle groups. Clearly the large muscles, because of their size, require more work than the small muscles. Moreover, the small muscles are often already involved when you work the large muscles. Along with the number of sets (see the preceding point), the number of exercises per muscle should reflect this difference.

Even at a high level, we advise you to do no more than three exercises per large muscle and no more than two exercises per small muscle.

Some people feel the need to constantly change their workouts. If this sounds like you, then feel free to do so. But most people like a routine and do not want to change exercises. This attitude is preferable for a beginner. Repeating the same exercises will improve your technique in performing the movements.

Basically, a muscle cannot give all its effort on a new exercise. There is a learning period where the muscle can learn to mobilize all its strength for a given movement. If you change your exercises too quickly, you do not have enough time to teach your muscles to really work hard during that movement. All the time spent learning a new exercise means a loss of time when you could be gaining muscle mass and improving your athletic performance. Constantly changing exercises when you do not need to will increase those nonproductive learning periods.

10. How many repetitions should you do in each set?

The number of repetitions is not the factor in your training program that will really determine the speed of your results. More than repetitions, what really counts is the intensity of the contraction. In general, you will gain more muscle mass when you perform 6 to 12 repetitions. But if you can do 15 repetitions at a given weight instead of the 12 that you envisioned, then do them! In the next set, however, you should increase the weight.

As a general rule, to gain strength without increasing muscle mass too much, you should do 1 to 4 repetitions.

For endurance, you must do at least 20 repetitions, and you could even go beyond 100.

Pyramid

Training a muscle can be explained using a pyramid. You must start with a light weight and a high number of repetitions (20, for example) to really warm up the muscle. In addition to warming up the muscle, this lets you work on the muscle's endurance.

For the second set, increase the weight enough so that you are targeting 12 repetitions. But as we said, do not stop during a set (except for warm-up) because you have reached your repetition goal.

For the third set, add weight so that you are targeting 8 repetitions. Here we have a good pyramid for the small muscle groups.

For the large groups, add more weight so that you are targeting 6 repetitions for a fourth set. For the fifth and sixth sets, you have the option to increase the weight (if you are mostly concerned about strength) or to decrease the weight to reach 15 to 20 repetitions (if you want more muscle mass or greater endurance).

For the last set, you can also alternate workouts where you lift more weight with workouts where you decrease the weight. In this way you have more rest days between two very intense workouts, which will speed your recovery time.

DEFINITION

The term **repetition** is the total number of times you perform a given movement in a set (see the definition of set on page 24). A repetition happens in three stages:

1. Positive stage—You lift the weight.
2. Static stage—You maintain the contracted position for one second.
3. Negative stage—You slowly lower the weight.

It is perfectly normal to wonder how many repetitions you should do in a set. But you should know that there is no magic number for repetitions.

11. How quickly should you perform repetitions?

As you have just seen, a repetition includes three distinct stages. To better learn how to master muscle contractions, it is best to start by moving the weight rather slowly.

The worst thing you can do as a beginner is to balance the weight and then use your body's momentum to lift the weight. This will create bad habits that are difficult to break later. At best, cheating will slow your progress. At worst, you will risk injuring yourself! When in doubt, lift the weight slowly rather than quickly.

> These basic rules do not apply to plyometric exercises, which must be as explosive as possible.

You should lift the weight using the muscle's strength and, therefore, slowly.

> - Take one or two seconds to lift the weight.
> - Hold the contracted position for one second while contracting the muscles as strongly as possible.
> - Slowly release and lower the weight over two seconds.

A repetition should take four to five seconds. If you go faster, you will not use the full strength of your muscles even if you lift a heavier weight.

Evolution

This is for basic technique. It is imperative that you master it perfectly before moving to a different strategy. After achieving good muscular control, you can increase the speed of each movement in order to achieve explosiveness. Explosiveness does not mean cheating. There is a very fine line between explosive training and losing control. This is why it is important to first master the muscle contraction before moving on to explosive movements.

An explosive repetition is suitable for the types of movements that are required in various sports. It is actually rare for a sport to require an athlete to move in a slow, controlled manner. In general, an athlete must move as quickly as possible. The goal of explosive training is to give you this speed.

The positive stage of an explosive repetition takes one half to one full second. There is no static stage, and the negative stage is done in half a second.

This type of repetition is more appropriate for athletes who are looking to improve performance than for people who want to develop muscle mass. People who want to develop muscle mass need to maintain slow, controlled movements. Remember also that poorly controlled explosive movements combined with heavy weights will hurt you rather than improve your performance.

Other techniques for altering the speed of your repetitions are available in the section titled Techniques for Increasing Intensity on page 41.

12. How long should a workout last?

The objective of a good workout is to stimulate muscles to their maximum in the shortest time possible. We are careful to favor a workout's intensity rather than its length.

The primary criteria that determine the duration of your workout are your schedule and your availability. If you do not have a lot of time, you should know that it is possible to do a complete workout in a short time—for example, with circuit training. For this, 15 to 20 minutes will suffice (see the section titled Techniques for Increasing Intensity on page 41 as well as section 3 of part 3 of this book). However, it is still preferable to allow at least 30 minutes for a workout.

Ideally, a good workout should last 45 minutes to a maximum of 60 minutes. If you spend more than 1 hour working out, this is a sign that your effort is not intense enough. At the end of 45 to 60 minutes, your muscles should be begging for mercy.

> A complete warm-up can take time, and this should not count against your 45- to 60-minute workout. For example, in the winter, you will need to increase your warm-up time. But the rest of your workout should not be cut short because your warm-up takes more time.

The duration of your workout will depend on two things:
1. Volume of work (number of exercises plus number of sets)
2. Rest time between sets

Rest time is the factor you need to adjust if you do not have enough time for your workout. We do not advise you to exercise for more than an hour because this means that you could

> - work too many muscles per session,
> - do too many exercises,
> - do too many sets, or
> - take too much rest time between sets.

16. Should you rest between working two muscle groups?

You are not required to take rest breaks between two muscle groups that you work during the same session. Catch your breath using the same amount of time you usually take between sets. You can increase the rest time if you feel fatigued, especially toward the end of your workout. However, you still need to keep doing the exercises rather quickly so that you stay warm and focused and so the session does not go on endlessly.

17. How do you pick the exercises that will work the best for you?

In this guide, we have carefully selected the most effective weight training exercises. They require practically no special equipment or perilous or precarious positions. However, all the exercises described may not necessarily suit you. Everyone has a different body type. Some people are large and some people are small. Some have broad shoulders and some have narrow shoulders. Every torso, leg, and arm is a different size.

To match different body types, you should choose exercises that work for you individually. We would be lying if we pretended that all body types could adapt to any exercise. Certain builds are just better suited for some exercises. Following are two examples that illustrate this concept of the difference between individuals and different exercises.

Unequal Difficulty

Since each person's body is different, some athletes will have an easier time than others. For example, a person with short arms will be able to do push-ups more easily because the range of motion is smaller. A person with very long arms will have a more difficult time because the range of motion is much greater. If their body weights are equal, then the long-armed person must move the same weight over a greater distance. It is a bit like one person who must run 100 yards while another person has to run only 90 yards in the same amount of time.

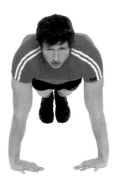
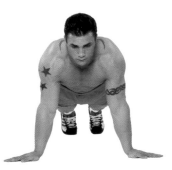

Unequal Danger

As a function of your body type, certain exercises could be more or less risky for you. As an example, when lifting weights in a squat, a person with long legs must lean farther forward than a person with short thighs. This is not about poor technique while performing an exercise. It is a question of body type. With short thighs, it is relatively easy to keep the back very straight. The longer your thighs are, the more you have to lean forward to maintain your balance. Unfortunately, the farther you lean forward, the greater chance you have of injuring your back.

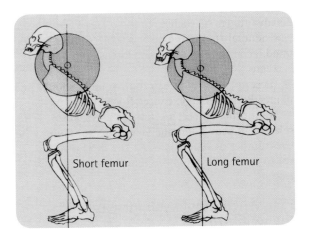

Short femur   Long femur

If body type should be taken into account when selecting an exercise, we note that in the specific description of the exercise.

There are two complementary ways to select your exercises:

1. By elimination. Some exercises do not work well with your anatomy. You should omit those. Other exercises do not match your goals. These two parameters will restrict the possibilities and, therefore, make your choices easier. However, simple elimination should not be your only criterion. It is better to find exercises that work for you.

2. By selection. To determine compatibility between your body type and an exercise, often the only way is to try the movement. You will find some exercises that you like right away. But most of the time you will find them a bit strange, and you will have difficulty performing them since they involve muscles that you are not accustomed to using. With time, the novelty will fade and you will feel the exercises more and more.

Learn to Differentiate Exercises

Your choice will be easier once you understand that there are differences between exercises. You should learn to recognize them and use them to your advantage. Thus, each exercise has advantages and disadvantages. Only by mastering this concept for each exercise will you find movements whose

> advantages most meet your needs, and
> disadvantages do not contradict your goals.

In part 2 of this book we are particularly attentive to describing the advantages and disadvantages of each movement. From there, you will have a solid and logical base from which to choose your exercises.

Before we describe the specific advantages and disadvantages of each exercise, we can highlight a few general things that you should always keep in mind.

There are two large categories of movements. Each of these two categories has strong points and weak points. By choosing exercises from one group rather than the other based on your needs, you will make the selection process that much easier.

Weight Training Exercises Can Be Divided Into Two Large Groups:

1 Multijoint exercises

These are exercises that work several joints at once. For example, the squat (bending the legs) forces you to move your knees, ankles, and hips. Three joints are made to work; therefore, this is a multijoint exercise. Determining whether or not an exercise belongs to the multijoint group is a secondary concern, right after you determine which muscles it uses.

ADVANTAGES

Multijoint exercises are more natural and more effective than isolation exercises (see page 32). In fact, muscles are made to work together and not one by one in an isolated manner. Multijoint exercises allow you to do the following:

> Stimulate a maximum number of muscle groups in a minimum amount of time.
> Manipulate heavy weights.
> Work within a range of motion where your muscles can easily express their full power.

- -

The popularity of multijoint movements should not overshadow their disadvantages:

> Because muscle mass comes into play, these are the hardest exercises physically. This is why many people avoid these exercises.
> Because of the number of muscles these exercises work, it is not always possible to target the muscles you wish to develop.

   For example, push-ups use the elbow and shoulder joints. Therefore, push-ups are a multijoint exercise. This movement works the chest, the shoulders, and the triceps. What is impossible to figure out is how much of the work each one of these muscles is performing. For some people, the chest muscles will do the majority of the work. Others will feel only their triceps contracting. Some people will feel it all in their shoulders. So recommending that someone do push-ups to build up the chest could be good advice or poor advice, depending on the individual. There is a random aspect to multijoint exercises that happens much less frequently with isolation exercises.

> In multijoint exercises, the range of motion is less than what a muscle can handle. This range does not necessarily correspond to the range that you need in your particular sport. On the other hand, when you have weak points that resist multijoint exercises, it is often because of the reduced range of motion with which they stimulate the muscle. In this case, only isolation exercises will provide you with the necessary range of motion.

DISADVANTAGES

Squat

Push-up

31

2 Isolation exercises

Isolation exercises include all movements that affect only one joint. For example, biceps curls (movement of the forearm over the arm) involve only the elbow joint. Even if this exercise is often described as a multijoint exercise for the arm, that description is technically incorrect.

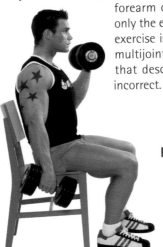

Flexing the arms

Chest fly

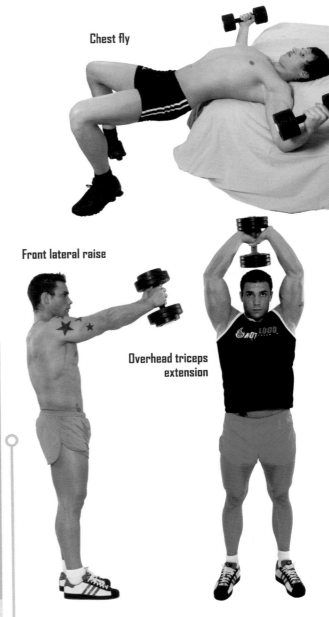

Front lateral raise

Overhead triceps extension

ADVANTAGES

> By using fewer muscle groups at one time, isolation exercises use less strength and energy. They are therefore much easier than multijoint exercises.
> Isolation exercises target muscles better than multijoint exercises. In general, it is difficult not to feel a muscle targeted by an isolation exercise.
> Isolation exercises are better for developing muscle control.
> If a muscle is not developing with the use of multijoint exercises, a few weeks of training with isolation exercises can wake it up. When you begin doing multijoint exercises again, you will feel that muscle working more. The muscle will then begin to respond to the work required by exercises that involve multiple joints.

- -

> Generally, isolation exercises are less effective than multijoint exercises in increasing strength and size.
> Muscle isolation is an artificial phenomenon. When you perform work requiring strength, your muscles are made to work together, not in an isolated fashion.
> If you tried to reproduce the work performed by multijoint exercises only with isolation exercises, you would waste a lot of time. For example, instead of doing a few push-ups, you would have to do a chest exercise plus a shoulder exercise plus a triceps exercise.
> The greater range of motion in isolation exercises does not allow you to use as heavy a weight as you would use in multijoint exercises.

DISADVANTAGES

Conclusion

Programs for beginners should primarily be made up of multijoint exercises. These allow for intense work on a maximum number of muscle groups in a minimum amount of time. Isolation exercises can later be added to these multijoint exercises in order to target certain areas that are delayed or that you really want to focus on.

Isolation exercises are secondary and are mainly for people searching to enhance appearance. In fact, as we have already seen, multijoint exercises do not necessarily stimulate all the muscles they are supposed to work in an equal manner. Certain groups will take precedence over others. Isolation exercises can help you maintain balance.

A State of Constant Evolution

As far as the choice of exercises goes, it is important not to get stuck in a rut. With time, you will realize that you are starting to appreciate exercises that you did not like before. When this happens, your first reaction might be regret that you did not realize it earlier. You might feel that you have lost some time. But this is rarely true. Muscle sensations are constantly changing. A month or two ago, your muscles were perhaps not ready for a certain exercise. The progress you have made means that you now feel more from that new exercise. So do not have any regrets.

The opposite can also happen: You feel less from an exercise that you really liked before. That exercise produced rapid progress at first, but it seems it has become ineffective. This is just a feeling.

Each of your movements has a very specific way of using the neuromuscular system. When you overwork a certain exercise, the neuromuscular system burns out. You lose sensations and the exercise becomes less effective. This means it is time to remove the exercise from your program. If you stop doing that exercise for several weeks, the neuromuscular system will be regenerated. You can then reintegrate the exercise into your program because it will once again allow you to make progress.

You must constantly adapt your neuromuscular system and not be rigid when faced with these changes. You might wonder how you will know when it is time to change your training program.

18. When should you change your training program?

Some people always prefer to repeat the same training program. This is easy to understand. After all, once you have found something that works, why change it? Other people constantly need new things. It is impossible to know which group you belong to, and most people are probably somewhere in between the two groups. But your state of mind reflects your muscles' needs fairly accurately. Two objective criteria demonstrate why you need to change your workout routine.

1. Plateau or regression in your strength. When your speed of progression abruptly stops, it means that something is no longer working. We are not talking about one or two workouts, but a tendency over at least two weeks. A radical change is required.

2. Boredom. When you lose your enthusiasm for exercising a certain muscle group or working out altogether, it means that your program is too monotonous. So you will need to make a change. But there are degrees of boredom that you must know how to interpret since they require varying degrees of change to your program. We begin with the kind of boredom that requires the most changes to your program and end with the kind of boredom that requires only slight alterations in your training program.

> **Severe boredom or even total lack of interest in working out.** This generally means you have been overtraining. It is time to take a break or reduce your volume of work. Restructuring your entire training will be beneficial.

> **Lack of interest for a given workout day.** This is a sign that you need to modify what you do on that specific day. Ask yourself if your lack of interest is related to the muscle groups you are working, the exercises you are doing, or the techniques you are using to increase intensity. Ask yourself the same question on the days you enjoy your workout the most. Why are you more motivated on those days? In other words, is there a way to transfer the enthusiasm from those days to the day when you are not excited about working out?

> **Lack of interest in working a given muscle.** Loss of interest in training a muscle that you enjoyed working out before is a strong indication that you need to change the exercises for that muscle. You do not need to change anything else for the rest of your body. You just need to change parts of the program for that muscle.

> **Lack of interest in an exercise.** As you saw in the previous point, lack of interest in an exercise that you liked before shows that you have burned out the specific neuromuscular structure for that movement. You should change the exercise in question before making any other changes.

Conclusion

There is no set rule for when you should change your program. As long as your program is giving you regular results in terms of gaining strength and increasing the number of repetitions, why change it? There will always come a time when you will feel the need to make changes. Your body will tell you by drastically reducing the pace of your progress. The difference between a beginner and an experienced athlete is the speed with which they perceive those signals. So be attentive and be sure to keep a notebook (see page 39) so that you can pick up on these clues quickly.

Also, on the days when you do not work out, take 30 seconds and hang from the pull-up bar just before you go to sleep. Being upright or sitting down during the day compresses the spine. This compression squeezes out the fluid inside each of your discs. This is why people are shorter in the evening than they are in the morning. But this fluid in your discs is required for good spinal health because it helps absorb shock. The loss of this fluid is at the heart of back pain. By hanging from the bar, you will gain recovery time, because a part of the spinal decompression that takes place during the night while lying down will already be done. The spine will recover better, and you will sleep better.

Waking up in the morning feeling that your spine remained compressed all night is the worst that can happen. This means that the lumbar muscles are not relaxed. Because of this nocturnal muscle tone, you sleep poorly, and you will quickly begin having frequent back pain. By relaxing the lumbar muscles and spine before going to sleep, you can avoid this very common problem.

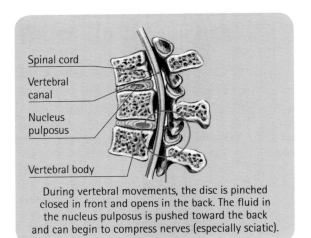

Spinal cord
Vertebral canal
Nucleus pulposus
Vertebral body

During vertebral movements, the disc is pinched closed in front and opens in the back. The fluid in the nucleus pulposus is pushed toward the back and can begin to compress nerves (especially sciatic).

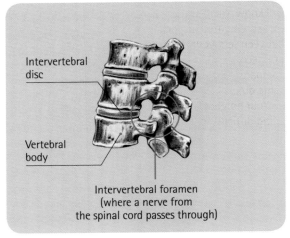

Intervertebral disc
Vertebral body

Intervertebral foramen (where a nerve from the spinal cord passes through)

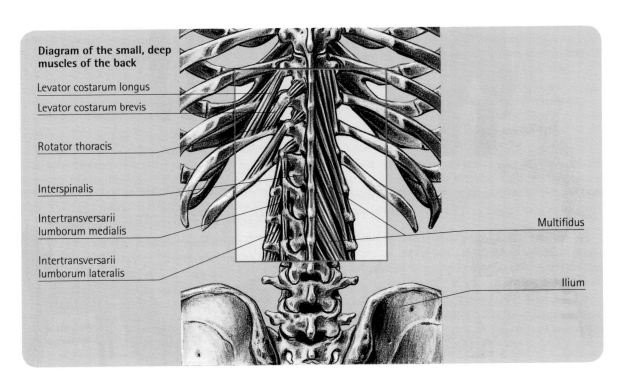

Diagram of the small, deep muscles of the back

Levator costarum longus
Levator costarum brevis
Rotator thoracis
Interspinalis
Intertransversarii lumborum medialis
Intertransversarii lumborum lateralis

Multifidus

Ilium

Tapering squats

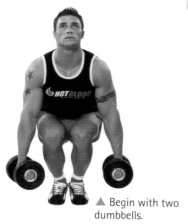

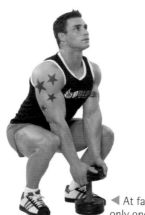

▲ Begin with two dumbbells.

◀ At failure, finish with only one dumbbell.

However, if you can continue your set by removing only a little bit of weight, this means your inroad is naturally weak. This is generally the case for beginners. Your inroad will increase with experience. In this specific case, it is important to train beyond failure.

> **NOTE**
> A tapering set that reaches a total of 20 repetitions (for example, 10 repetitions to failure, then tapering plus 5 repetitions to failure again, then tapering again plus 5 repetitions, then failure again) is very different from a normal set of 20 repetitions. If the final number of repetitions is the same in both cases, then tapering has allowed you to do the following:
> - ➤ Begin the set with a weight that was much too heavy.
> - ➤ Reach failure three times instead of one time.
> Handling heavy weights and pushing your muscles to failure force the muscle to grow. Tapering is a very effective technique for this.

Example of a rest break

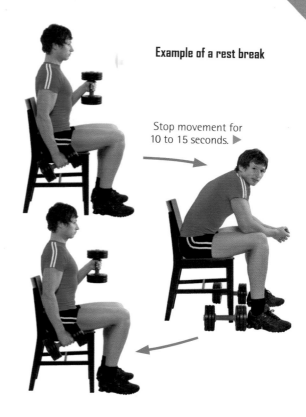

Stop movement for 10 to 15 seconds. ▶

Rest Break

When you reach failure, stop the movement for 10 to 15 seconds to give your muscle a break. After this brief pause, begin your set again.

The goal is to do one or two extra repetitions. Rest breaks are often used with very heavy weights. You do the maximum or a double repetition before stopping briefly to catch your breath. Then, try a repetition and so on until the rest break does not allow you to gather enough strength to do one more repetition.

Beginners who have difficulty with pull-ups can also use this technique. If you can lift yourself only one or two times, take a 10- to 30-second break at failure, and try again. Soon the break will become unnecessary and you will be able to keep doing repetitions.

When you are doing very long sets, it is common to take a rest break without really being aware of it in order to catch your breath and do even more repetitions.

The rest break somewhat resembles a stop-and-go (see page 48), but it has a completely different objective. Stopping the movement is done for a longer period and, if possible, is not done just before the contraction phase.

Negatives

Negatives are also called eccentric repetitions. The negative effort involves the part of the exercise when you lower the weight or your body. It is the opposite of the positive effort, which involves lifting the weight or your body weight.

For example, when you are climbing stairs, you are basically working your quads positively. However, when you go down those same stairs, your muscles are working negatively. They are only slowing down or stopping your body. Imagine that two people are faced with a set of very steep stairs. One person must descend the stairs and the other must climb them. It is much more tiring to climb up the stairs. However, it is more perilous to descend the stairs since you will gain speed as you go down. Your muscles, working in a negative mode, will slow you down, stopping you from gaining too much speed and falling.

What is surprising with eccentric repetitions is that in the days that follow, the person who descended the stairs will have the most aches and pains. In fact, even if the negative effort appears to be easier on a muscle, it is also the most traumatic for it. All the tiny stretches that the muscle does to slow you down cause damage to the muscle cells. The body has to react to this trauma by increasing its strength and developing its volume. This is why scientific research shows without question that working negatively is more productive than working positively for gaining muscle mass and strength. To continue with the stairs example, the person who descends the stairs every day for one month will end up with stronger thighs than the person who only climbs the stairs.

Conclusion

The negative part of an exercise takes on special significance for your progress. You should pay particular attention to it so that you can ensure optimal development of your muscles. There are five different but complementary ways to use this physiological property of your muscles.

1 **Slowing down the descent on each repetition**
When you begin the negative phase of a weight training exercise, you can do the following:

> Let the weight go without trying to hold it.
> Or, on the other hand, try to slow it down using the strength of your muscles.

A typical example of the first case is Olympic weightlifting. In weightlifting there is almost no negative effort. Weightlifters lift the bar, and once they have performed the movement, they let the bar go without trying to slow it down.

But in most sports, there is a negative phase. A typical example is skiing. Contrary to popular belief, skiers' muscles do not work in a static manner. Their quads are constantly trying to slow down on the ruggedness of the slope. Negative work is particularly important in this case.

Athletes must also analyze the role of negative strength in their sports. The more important it is for their performance, the more they should work at it during weight training.

2 **Role of negative phase in increasing muscle mass**
For those who want to gain muscle mass, the negative phase is more important than the positive phase. The descent of the weight must therefore be systematically slowed down. However, slowing it down in the negative phase should be done gradually. For example, in a set with eight repetitions, slow down briefly only on the first three repetitions. Since it is easier to slow down a weight than to lift it, it would be too easy (and inefficient) to act too soon on the negative phase. However, as you do repetitions, your muscles get more tired and you will then start slowing down in the negative phase. During the last few repetitions, the weight must be lowered as slowly as possible.

> **NOTE**
> You should always finish a movement in the negative phase, not the positive phase. For example, when doing push-ups, there is a natural tendency to want to end with your arms extended. But instead, you should stop when you are lying on the floor and you cannot push up any more. The negative movement that brought you to the floor should have been very slow and controlled with all your strength.

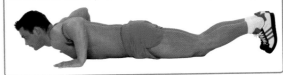

One mistake to avoid is to hold the weight for 5 or 10 seconds at the top of a movement before letting it fall with no control. Slowing down does not mean stopping. Let the weight stretch your muscles by slowing down more and more with every repetition.

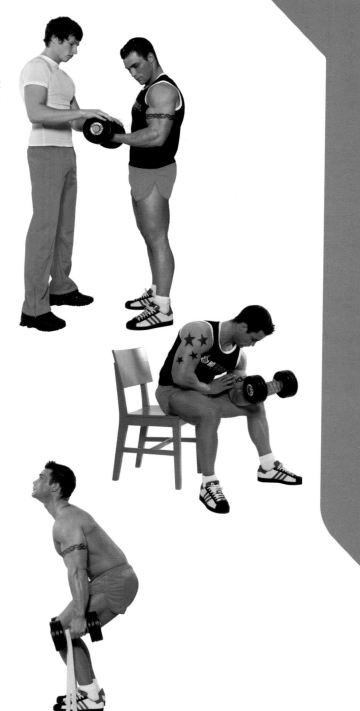

3 Accentuating resistance during the descent

The negative strength of a muscle is more important than the positive strength. If you can lift 45 pounds with one arm, you could probably hold back 65 pounds. So an ideal set should contain a negative done with more weight than the positive to achieve maximum results. There are three ways to disassociate the negative weight from the positive weight. Use one of them during every second or third workout.

1. Work with a partner. The easiest way is to work out with a partner who can push the weight or push on your body to accentuate the weight during the return phase of the movement. Unfortunately, people rarely work out with a partner. But you can manage without one.

2. Use your free hand. Working out one side at a time (see page 50) allows you to keep one hand free. This hand can often be used to accentuate the weight of the arm that is working during the negative phase. For example, with concentration curls for the biceps, you lift the dumbbell normally. When you release the weight, you push on the dumbbell so that you add 10 to 20 pounds.

3. Use an elastic band. As we explained in the section on choosing your equipment, elastic bands have unique resistance properties. When you pull on a band, it accumulates elastic energy (or strength). When you let go, it will immediately return to its normal shape. In weight training, a band provides an acceleration of the negative phase that no other equipment can provide. This is the main advantage of bands: They progressively accumulate a large amount of tension. This tension will be reproduced abruptly in the negative phase. The muscles have to work much more intensely than with traditional weights to slow down the band's resistance. This challenge results in a faster gain in strength, power, and muscle mass than with traditional weights.

This is why, for about 10 years, more and more athletic teams in the United States (in particular, American football players) have been attaching bands to the weights they lift. This technique is still relatively unknown in Europe.

NOTE
Through the intermediary of your muscles (which act similar to elastic bands), a portion of the tension in the band accumulates in the muscles during the negative phase. This strength coming from outside will be used by your muscles to lift the weight. In other words, not only is the negative phase accentuated when using bands, but bands also allow the muscles to become immediately stronger and lift heavier weights because of the external assistance they provide. There is a double benefit, which explains the popularity of this method in American sports.

4 Pure negatives

To be able to do your maximum in the negative, the positive phase is eliminated. The movement consists of just struggling against gravity with as heavy a weight as possible. This technique is particularly appropriate when you do not have enough strength to do pull-ups, for example. In this case, you always have enough strength to slow down the descent. The goal is to slow down the descent for as long as possible and as many times as possible. The magic of pure negatives is that they allow you to quickly gain enough strength to be able to lift your body alone. In general, two weeks of pure negative training at the pull-up bar will allow a person who was not capable of doing a pull-up to do a pull-up once or twice all by himself.

Another technique is to lift the weight with two arms but to lower it with only one arm. For example, when doing push-ups, lift yourself up normally with two arms. Once you are up, transfer your weight to one arm and do a pure negative. Be sure that you are at an adequate level of fitness before attempting this variation. If you cannot stop yourself, especially at the end, you can do a partial negative. This means descending part of the way and then going back up using both arms. Your strength will quickly increase and you will be able to go down all the way without any problems.

Numerous movements (but not all of them) lend themselves to pure negatives. Use this strategy at least once a month.

5 Postfailure negatives

To go beyond failure, you can adopt a strategy that is a little different. For example, do as many push-ups as you can. At failure, get back up using your legs so that you can reposition yourself with your arms extended. From there, lower yourself slowly. Once you are on the floor, get back up using your legs, and then repeat the move for a pure negative. This same strategy can be used at the pull-up bar, where you push on the floor or on a chair to get back up into the position for contraction.

Stop-and-Go

This technique involves pausing for one second between the negative phase of the exercise and the contraction.

For example, when doing push-ups, you stay elongated on the floor for one second. You relax the muscles and then activate them, causing the contraction. The goal of this pause is to eliminate the accumulation of elastic energy that took place during the negative phase of the exercise.

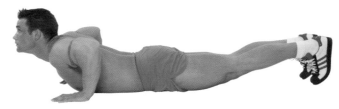

This strategy has three practical applications:

1 It is useful in disciplines that require a lot of strength at the initial stage, as in sprints. In this case, the muscles need to contract as powerfully as possible without having been prestretched. So they are relatively weak while you are forcing them to be immediately powerful. This is a physical quality that you can develop using the stop-and-go technique.

2 Stop-and-go alters the structure of how muscles are harnessed. For example, when doing push-ups normally, you can really feel the work in your chest, but not so much in your triceps. By pausing just before the contraction phase, you might be able to overturn this feeling. Many people will feel a different kind of muscular work, which could be oriented more toward the triceps, for example. So, if an exercise is not correctly targeting a muscle that it is supposed to work, give it a second chance by trying it with the stop-and-go method.

3 Certain fragile joints cannot really handle the pressure generated on the tendons at the moment when the exercise goes from an eccentric phase to a concentric phase. This transition can be softened with the pause provided by the stop-and-go method.

Absolutely all exercises can be done with the stop-and-go method. This variation will produce benefits with certain movements, but not with all of them. It is up to you to test it out and determine for yourself which exercises work best with this pause.

Burn

When lactic acid accumulates in your muscles during a set, it is referred to as burn.

This burning means that it is difficult for the muscle to maintain the intensity of the effort you are demanding. It is a signal for muscular overload.

As with pain, burn is an obstacle to performance. The goal with burn is to turn the obstacle around and do it with strength. Instead of avoiding the burn, you will try to create it since it means there is stimulation that will force the muscle to grow larger. Once you have generated burn, the challenge is to try to put up with it for as long as possible before quitting.

In general, burn appears after 12 intense repetitions. So going for burn is something you do with lighter weights. Continuous tension, supersets (see page 51), and tapering are good ways to test your will when facing burn.

Continuous Tension

One of the ways to increase the difficulty of an exercise without increasing the weight is to maintain continuous tension in the muscle. This means that at no time during the movement will you let the muscle relax or "breathe."

For example, while doing push-ups, when you hover with your arms extended, your skeleton is supporting the weight of your body and not your muscles. In this position, your muscles can recover somewhat.

The principle of continuous tension means eliminating the phase where the arms (or the legs) are extended. The whole time you are doing push-ups, you keep your arms slightly bent. An intense burn will quickly develop in the muscle because of the intracellular asphyxiation you are creating. In effect, by constantly keeping the muscles under tension, you are blocking the circulation of blood. Without oxygen, the muscles produce a lot of waste (lactic acid) when they synthesize their energy.

The same principle applies to the shoulders, back, biceps, or triceps: You never straighten your arms during the exercise. For the quads, you never completely straighten the portion of your legs above the knees. Ideally, you should use a mixture: continuous tension and rest break. You begin the movement with continuous tension. When the pain becomes too much to bear, you take a break (arms or legs straight) so that some of the lactic acid can leave the muscles. The exercise can then continue for one or two additional repetitions.

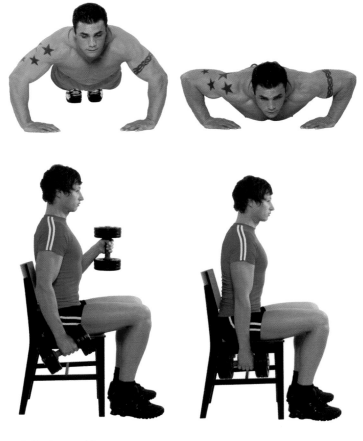

▲ Begin set without straight arms.

▲ At end of set, rest with arms straight to get a few extra repetitions.

49

Unilateral Training

Most weight training exercises are done bilaterally, which means contracting the muscles on both the left and the right sides.

This symmetry of movement is not found in everyday gestures, though. Like walking or running, most of your movements are unilateral. You contract the muscles on only one side of the body at a time. Humans are unilateral beings. We are the opposite of rabbits, because they use two of their feet simultaneously to move forward. Humans move forward one foot at a time, using unilateral muscle work.

Humans' natural tendency toward unilateralism explains why strength is about 10 percent greater when we work unilaterally rather than bilaterally. If you can do biceps curls with a maximum of 110 pounds using both arms simultaneously, then unilaterally, the sum of both arms (what you can lift with the right arm, then what you can lift with the left arm) will not be 110 pounds, but about 121 pounds.

There is a loss of effectiveness in the central nervous system during bilateral work. One way to see this is to do dumbbell curls. Start the exercise contracting both arms at the same time. At failure, you can probably get one or two additional repetitions if you contract the right biceps while letting the left arm hang straight. This gain in strength is brought about by the increase in effectiveness of the central nervous system when you contract only one side at a time.

However, unilateral training is not always easy to do. For example, it is difficult to do push-ups or pull-ups with only one arm at a time. But you can find unilateral exercises for every muscle. This is a characteristic that we specify for each exercise in part 2 of this book.

There are two variations of unilateral training:

1 Alternating unilateral training

In the example of the curls, you contract the right biceps. Only when the right arm returns to its starting position does the left arm begin its work.

The advantage of this technique is that the right arm can rest while the left arm works. The disadvantage is that the nerve impulses must constantly shift back and forth between the left and the right, which is not ideal. However, certain sports require this criss-cross (for example, running or swimming the crawl). If this is the case in your sport, this particularity should be a part of your weight training exercises so that your nervous system is well prepared for this difficulty. If not, you can choose the second variation.

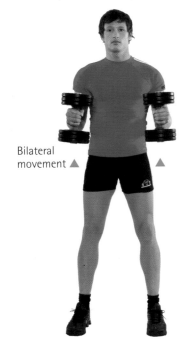

Bilateral movement ▲   ▲

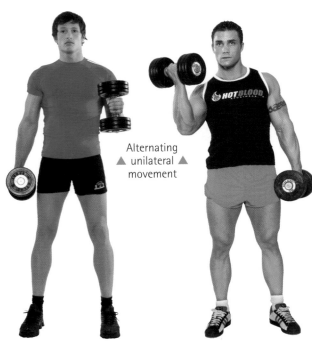

Alternating
▲ unilateral ▲
movement

50

2 Pure unilateral training

In this version, only one side of the body is worked out. You do an entire set with the muscles on the right side.

Pure unilateral training ▶

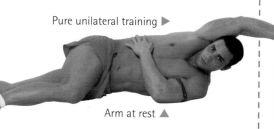

Arm at rest ▲

You rest a bit before doing your set with the muscles on the left side. Again, you take a small rest before returning to the right side. The central nervous system can express its full power in this configuration. The contraction as well as the concentration on the working muscles will be at their maximum. Athletes whose sport requires such work (shot put, for example) should use this technique generously. Pure unilateral training often offers the unique advantage of allowing you to do accentuated negatives and forced repetitions with your free hand.

The disadvantage of this technique is that it increases the overall workout time, because you are doubling the number of sets that you need to do.

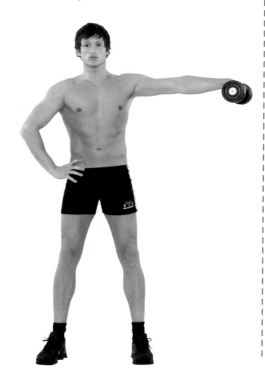

2 Supersets for the same muscl

You do two exercises in a row for t
The objective is to increase th
These supersets are simil
changing the exercise
weight than the first
the set beyond fa

There are t
1. Cl
mult
is

There are two kinds of supersets:

1 Antagonistic muscle supersets

This is where you do an exercise for one muscle and then immediately do another exercise for the opposing muscle. The most popular superset is where you combine a biceps exercise with a triceps exercise. These are the other antagonistic supersets:

> Chest and back
> Front shoulders and rear shoulders
> Abdomen and low back
> Quadriceps and hamstrings

The main advantage of this strategy is that it saves you time. In effect, it is no longer necessary to rest between sets. The biceps will recover while the triceps is working. The triceps will rest when you work the biceps. In addition to improving your strength, your endurance will improve.

51

...ne biceps, for example. ...e intensity of the effort. ...ar to tapering but involve ...The second exercise uses less ...t, which means you can continue ...ure.

...ree kinds of supersets for the same muscle:
...ssic superset. This superset includes either two ...joint exercises or two isolation exercises. The goal ...imply to do two exercises in a row so that you go beyond failure.

The sophistication of the other two variations of supersets explains why they are more popular than classic supersets.

2. Preexhaustion superset. The exercises for this superset are used in a very particular way. You must begin with an isolation exercise followed by a multijoint exercise. The goal is to tire the target muscle with the isolation exercise. During the multijoint exercise, the target muscle continues to work, despite fatigue, with the help of the other muscle groups.

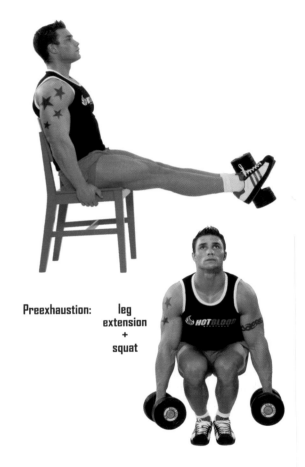

Preexhaustion: leg extension + squat

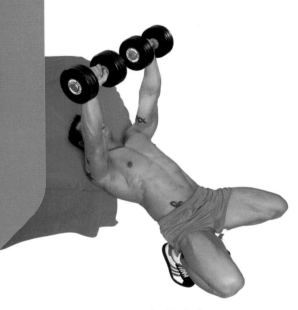

Classic superset: dumbbell chest press + push-up

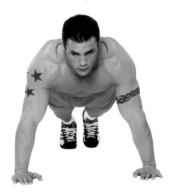

The theoretical justification for preexhaustion is that in most multijoint exercises, the target muscle does not tire out first; rather, the other small adjoining muscles tire out first. Thus, when you are doing push-ups, fatigue in your chest muscles is not what stops you; fatigue in your triceps stops you. Because of this lack of strength in your arms, the chest did not have enough time to really work. Because they reach exhaustion first, the triceps limit your ability to stimulate your chest muscles. This is why you will prework and tire out the chest muscles using an isolation movement before beginning push-ups.

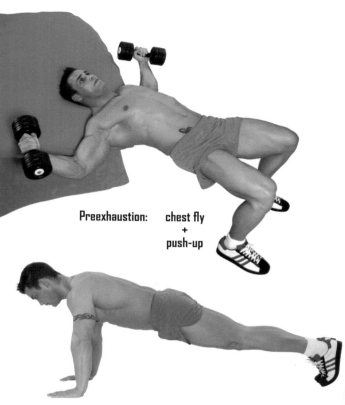

Preexhaustion: **chest fly**
+
push-up

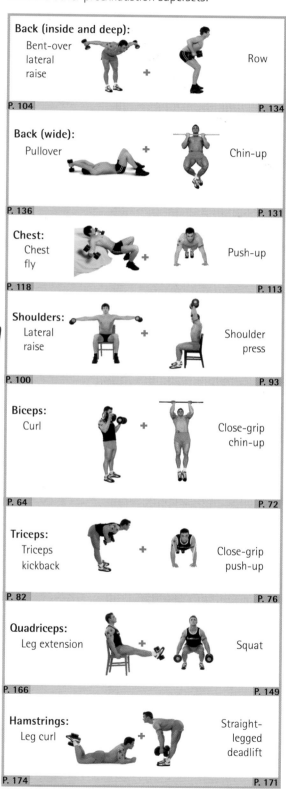

Here are other preexhaustion supersets:

Back (inside and deep):
Bent-over lateral raise + Row
P. 104 — P. 134

Back (wide):
Pullover + Chin-up
P. 136 — P. 131

Chest:
Chest fly + Push-up
P. 118 — P. 113

Shoulders:
Lateral raise + Shoulder press
P. 100 — P. 93

Biceps:
Curl + Close-grip chin-up
P. 64 — P. 72

Triceps:
Triceps kickback + Close-grip push-up
P. 82 — P. 76

Quadriceps:
Leg extension + Squat
P. 166 — P. 149

Hamstrings:
Leg curl + Straight-legged deadlift
P. 174 — P. 171

The principle applies not only to the chest muscles but also to all other large muscle groups. For example, for the shoulders, you should do the lateral raise followed by the shoulder press. The lateral raise will have fatigued the deltoid muscles. The deltoids will be supported during the work of the shoulder press by a portion of the pectoralis major and the triceps.

Preexhaustion can also help you to better feel a muscle that you have difficulty working. If you have problems feeling your pectoralis major muscles while doing push-ups, then doing an isolation exercise beforehand allows you to burn the chest muscles a bit so that you will feel them immediately during push-ups.

! This is only theory. Preexhaustion can unfortunately prove to be counterproductive. In the example of shoulder work, it often happens that the triceps do all the work during the shoulder press because the deltoids have been so worn out by the lateral raises that they have no strength to assist in the multijoint exercise. This explains why you feel the fatigue in the triceps instead of the shoulders.

3. Postexhaustion superset. The logic of post-exhaustion is exactly the opposite of preexhaustion. The goal is to work the target muscle to the maximum using a multijoint exercise. At failure, you move to an easier isolation exercise, which allows the target muscle to give everything it has left. In the shoulder example, you give everything you have during the shoulder press. You do not have to worry if fatigue in the triceps forces you to stop the movement, since you are going to go at it again with an isolation exercise that targets only the deltoids.

Postexhaustion lets you know you have really worn out the targeted muscle. Postexhaustion supersets are exactly the inverse of those listed for preexhaustion.

Postexhaustion: shoulder press + lateral raise

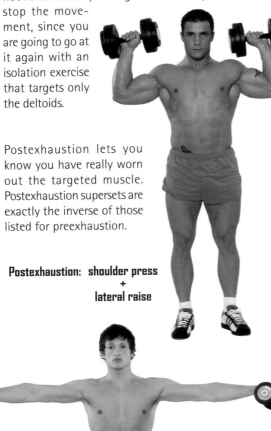

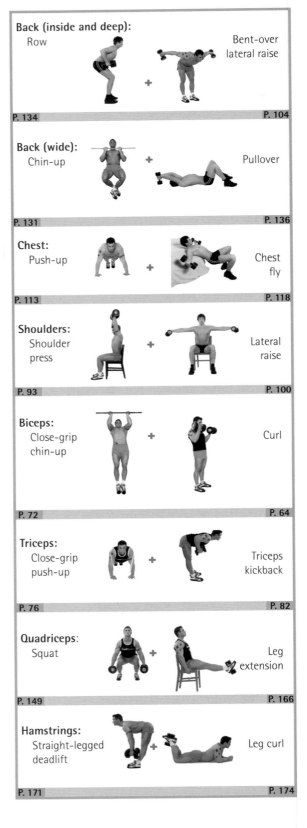

Back (inside and deep):
Row   Bent-over lateral raise

P. 134   P. 104

Back (wide):
Chin-up   Pullover

P. 131   P. 136

Chest:
Push-up   Chest fly

P. 113   P. 118

Shoulders:
Shoulder press   Lateral raise

P. 93   P. 100

Biceps:
Close-grip chin-up   Curl

P. 72   P. 64

Triceps:
Close-grip push-up   Triceps kickback

P. 76   P. 82

Quadriceps:
Squat   Leg extension

P. 149   P. 166

Hamstrings:
Straight-legged deadlift   Leg curl

P. 171   P. 174

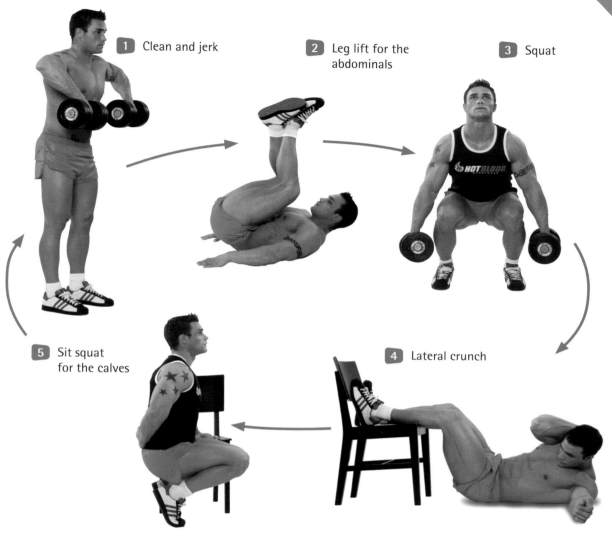

1 Clean and jerk

2 Leg lift for the abdominals

3 Squat

5 Sit squat for the calves

4 Lateral crunch

Circuits

Circuits are mostly used by athletes who want to increase functional strength or by people who want muscular or cardiorespiratory training. Circuits also make for shorter workouts because not much rest time is involved.

With classic weight training, the workouts for each muscle were separated artificially. You did several sets of an exercise for one muscle group (chest, for example) before moving to a new muscle (such as the back). But the body is not made to work this way. In most sports, the muscles have to work together.

While in certain disciplines you repeat the same movement (running, swimming, etc.), in others you must do combinations of very different movements. For example, in rugby, you run forward, backward, and to the side, and you push with your arms.

Circuits are most appropriate for these kinds of sports that require you to constantly change your movements. In fact, the continual changes in circuit exercises are closer to what is required on the field than a classic weight training workout.

In addition, the circuit develops endurance coupled with strength much more than working in sets can. Circuits are therefore indicated for sports that require strength and endurance. However, circuits do not have much of an advantage (except for saving time) when muscle mass is the primary goal. Circuits are described in detail in part 3.

How Should You Breathe While Exercising?

Your breathing will affect your performance.

> - Muscles can demonstrate their full power only when respiration is blocked.
> - They are a little weaker when you exhale.
> - They are at their weakest when you inhale.

These physiological reactions are perfectly illustrated by the strategy adopted by arm wrestling champions. They wait until the opponent inhales and then hold their breath and use all their strength to win. In other words, they gather all their strength by holding their breath at the moment their opponent is at his weakest because he is inhaling.

You should use these particularities to your advantage. In general, weight training books recommend that you not hold your breath. This is because those books are written by people who have never worked out intensely before. Holding your breath is a natural reflex. Strength, reaction time, precision of the movement, and concentration are briefly improved while the breath is held. Another advantage of holding your breath is that it tightens the spinal column. In this way, breath holding protects the back when the spinal column is subjected to great pressure.

A study done among elite sprinters showed that all champion athletes hold their breath when the starting gun goes off. When researchers asked them why, 91 percent of them said that they held their breath on purpose. When the scientists verified the behavior of the other 9 percent, they discovered that those sprinters held their breath as well, even though they were not aware of it.

▌Problems With Holding Your Breath
Even if muscular power increases, there are still two inherent problems with holding your breath.

1. Cardiac risk. When you hold your breath, you are doing a Valsalva maneuver. This apnea puts a certain pressure on your heart. This is perfectly fine for people in good health. However, for someone with cardiac problems, breath holding is not recommended because it could be dangerous.

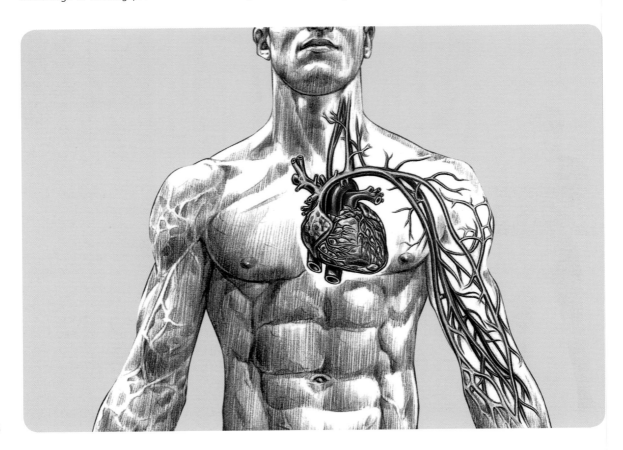

Breathe in the best you can between repetitions or during the easiest phase of the movement (the descent of the weight). Contrary to inspiration, which must be forced, expiration comes naturally at the moment when muscle pressure is reduced somewhat. But the difficulty in getting enough air during a hard set explains why this type of effort results in shortness of breath.

Good breathing in weight training is a technique that you must learn. It is much less simple than it seems. It will take time before you completely master it, but it will ultimately help you progress.

2. More rapid fatigue. When you hold your breath, you asphyxiate even more quickly since it happens at the moment the muscle is acting with its full strength. The longer you hold your breath during each repetition, the more quickly you become tired.

▌Breathing During Heavy Work
The more you plan to work with heavy weights, the more you need to take advantage of breath holding to optimize your performance. What you must do in order to avoid the problems we have described is to hold your breath

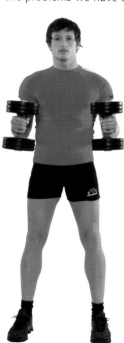

for as short a time as possible. This brief instance of breath holding should come exactly when the movement is the hardest. For example, when you work the biceps and are bringing your hands toward your shoulders, the moment when the forearms are parallel to the ground is the hardest. Before and after this angle, the movement is easier. It would be counterproductive to hold your breath the entire time you are lifting the weight. You need to do it for just a fraction of a second when the forearms reach parallel position. On the contrary, what you must not do is inhale at that particular moment. In the worst case, exhale!

▌Breathing During Light Endurance Exercise
When the work is light or long, you must breathe as much as possible to avoid depriving muscles of oxygen. In this case, it is better to avoid holding your breath, despite the natural tendency to do so. Exhale during the most difficult part of the exercise (lifting the weight or the body) and inhale during the easiest part (lowering the weight).

▌Breathing During Plyometric Exercise
Breath holding must occur when you contact the floor so that your muscles are more rigid and you get a better rebound. The body will block respiration more or less on its own without your interference. Training will offer you shorter breath-holding periods that do not deprive the muscles of oxygen for as long, and you will be better synchronized with the maximum muscular effort.

▌Breathing During Stretching
When stretching, the logic of breathing is reversed. To stretch, you must relax the muscle. Holding your breath during a stretch will make the muscle more rigid. So you must inhale so that the muscle will become less rigid and stretch farther.

▌Breathing Between Sets
During rest breaks, you must work on your breathing. Do not hyperventilate and end up dizzy. The ideal would be to go to a window and breathe calmly.

▌Conclusion
As far as breathing is concerned, you do not have to prove anything. Above all, you should be concerned about efficiency.

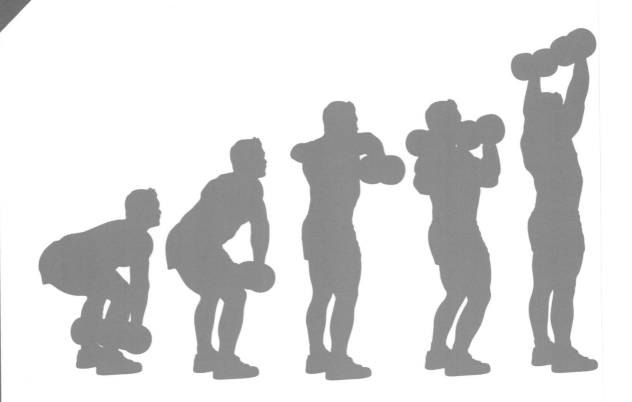

PART 2

Exercises

59

STRENGTHEN YOUR ARMS

The arm is divided into three large muscle groups: biceps, triceps, and forearm.

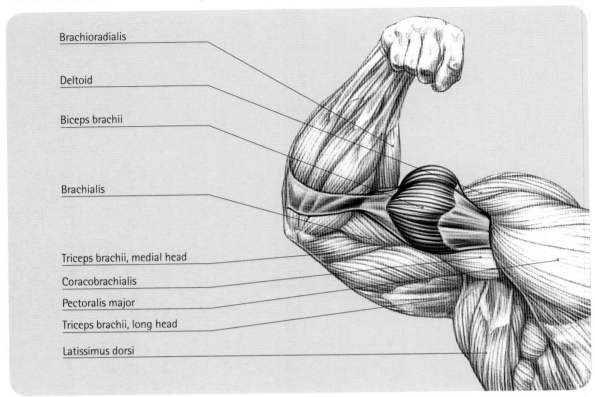

- Brachioradialis
- Deltoid
- Biceps brachii
- Brachialis
- Triceps brachii, medial head
- Coracobrachialis
- Pectoralis major
- Triceps brachii, long head
- Latissimus dorsi

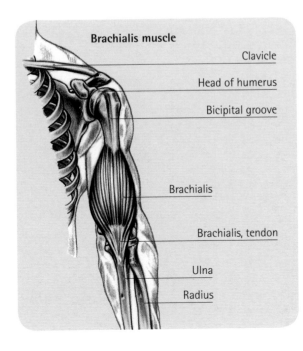

Brachialis muscle
- Clavicle
- Head of humerus
- Bicipital groove
- Brachialis
- Brachialis, tendon
- Ulna
- Radius

Biceps

▌Role of the Biceps

The arms, the biceps in particular, are the standard indication of a muscular physique. Usually most people want to develop the biceps first. Outside of its purely aesthetic role, the job of the biceps is to flex the forearm and lift it toward the upper arm.

To develop powerful arms quickly, you need to understand that the biceps is not alone; it is assisted by two other muscles:

1. The brachialis muscle. This muscle is located underneath the biceps and is somewhat like a second biceps. The brachialis muscle has the potential to become as large as the biceps. But this rarely happens! This is good news because it means there are easy inches to gain by specifically focusing on this muscle. The reason the brachialis is not usually well developed is that it is difficult to work this muscle with weight training exercises since it is not often used for daily activities.

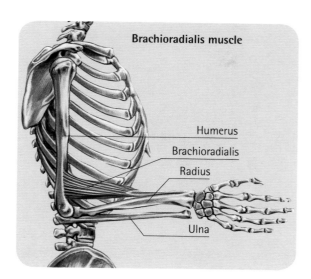

Brachioradialis muscle

Humerus

Brachioradialis

Radius

Ulna

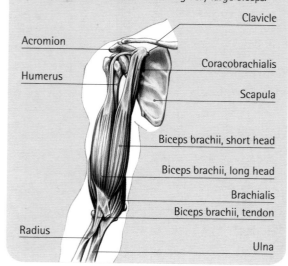

Of the two heads (parts of the muscle) that make up the biceps, the long head (the one on the exterior) is the most visible. The short head (the internal part of the biceps) is somewhat hidden by the torso. The long head is the part you should emphasize so you can quickly create the illusion of having very large biceps.

Clavicle

Acromion

Coracobrachialis

Humerus

Scapula

Biceps brachii, short head

Biceps brachii, long head

Brachialis

Biceps brachii, tendon

Radius

Ulna

2. The brachioradialis muscle. Technically, this muscle belongs to the forearm. But the brachioradialis muscle creates a good part of the arm's thickness. Without it, you could have big arms, but they would not be impressive. Even if it does not add an inch to your arm circumference, a chiseled brachioradialis muscle makes it look like you have powerful arms.

Only the harmonious development of these three muscles will make your biceps look really impressive.

Three Hand Positions

Basically, the hand can be placed in three different positions.

1 Neutral position

The thumb is pointing up. The arm is strongest when the hand is in this position. However, the biceps is not in the ideal position to demonstrate its full power. In this position, the brachioradialis and the radialis muscles provide most of the arm's strength.

2 Supination

The pinkie finger is close to your body and the thumb is away from your body so that your palm is facing up. This is the best position for working the biceps.

3 Pronation

The thumb is close to your body and the pinkie finger is away from your body so that your palm is facing down. This is the weakest position for the arm. Work is primarily done by the brachioradialis muscle, while the biceps cannot be of much help.

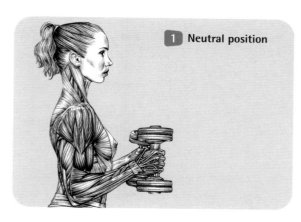

1 Neutral position

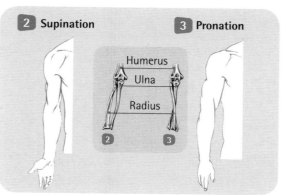

2 Supination

3 Pronation

Humerus

Ulna

Radius

61

The biceps, a part of the triceps, the calves, the hamstrings, and the quadriceps are multijoint muscles. This means that they attach to two joints at the same time. The chest, shoulders, and back muscles are single-joint muscles; they attach to only one joint. Multijoint muscles are very powerful. They are so strong because their length does not have to change much during an exercise. Unlike single-joint muscles, they can take advantage of the length–tension relationship.

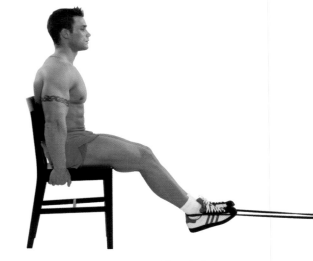

One example of maintaining optimal length during an exercise: a seated leg curl for the hamstrings.

▌A Muscle's Length–Tension Relationship: The Secret to Strength

A muscle's strength is unequal along its length. The more stretched (lengthened) a muscle is, the more it loses its ability to generate force. In the same way, the more a muscle is shortened (contracted), the more it loses strength. It is between these two extreme positions that it can produce the most tension. This is the muscle's optimal length. The relationship between a muscle's length and its ability to generate force is called the length–tension relationship.

The length–tension relationship is not so important for single-joint muscles. In fact, you cannot use this relationship with single-joint muscles because when you contract a single-joint muscle, it always gets shorter. However, it is very important to use the length–tension relationship when working multijoint muscles. With these muscles, it is possible to do the following:

> ➤ Shorten the muscle at both ends. In this case, the muscle will be relatively weak.

> ➤ Shorten the muscle at one end while lengthening the other end. In these conditions, a multijoint muscle can express its full power. In fact, since it is stretched at one end and contracted at the other, it is at a length that is close to its optimum. That is the length where it can generate the most force.

As an example, this is what happens with the biceps during a pull-up: The biceps shortens where it attaches to the forearm. However, it lengthens where it attaches to the shoulder.

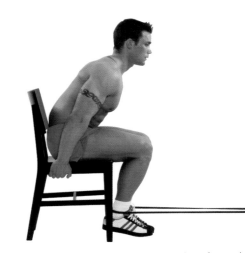

By contracting the muscles, you begin to lean forward to stretch your thighs.

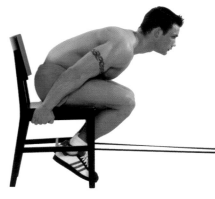

You continue to lean forward. The result: You bring the feet under the body while the length of the hamstrings has not changed much.

ARMS

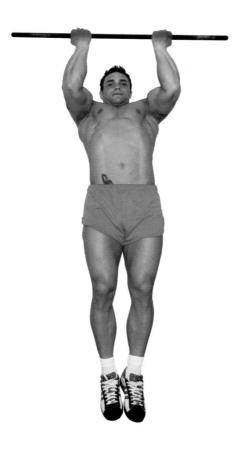

In general, multijoint exercises use this physiological property of double-joint muscles. This is why they are more effective than isolation exercises, which can only shorten the muscle. In fact, muscles develop more easily when they are worked at a length that is close to their optimum.

Applications for Sports

In running, the muscles for movement are primarily multijoint muscles (the hamstrings, calves, and rectus femoris). If they were single-joint muscles, then you would not be able to run very far for very long. Mother Nature knew what she was doing.

For example, the hamstrings lengthen near the glutes and shorten near the knee when the thigh moves forward. When the leg returns and goes backward, the hamstrings contract near the glutes and lengthen near the knee. Since the muscles maintain a length close to their optimum, you are able to move efficiently.

The length–tension relationship of multijoint muscles is a property that you must absolutely use if you want to quickly gain strength and size. For each muscle you work, you need to determine whether it is a multijoint muscle. For multijoint muscles, you should know if you are doing a multijoint exercise (which makes the most of the relationship) or an isolation exercise (which prevents you from taking advantage of the relationship). This is important information that we provide at the beginning of each exercise page.

The biceps is a shining example of this physiological characteristic.

One of my arms is longer than the other!
It is normal that you are not perfectly symmetrical. No one is, so try not to worry about it.
Size matters.
Impressive arms start at about 16 inches (40 cm) in diameter. Really impressive arms measure from 18 to 18.5 inches (45.5–47 cm). Abnormal measurements beyond these are very difficult to attain unless you are already a very large person.

/// Supinated Curl

This exercise works the biceps in particular, but it also works the brachialis and brachioradialis muscles to some degree. It is an isolation exercise, not a multijoint exercise, since only one joint (the elbow) is involved. Working unilaterally is better if large biceps are your primary goal.

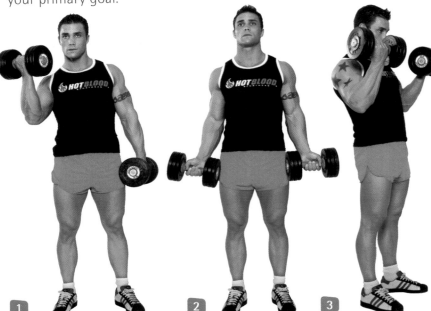

! If you cheat too much by swinging your torso from front to back so that you can use a heavier weight or do a few more repetitions, you are risking an injury to your back. To learn to do the exercise perfectly, you can begin by doing it with your back against the wall.

1 Hold your hand in a neutral position and then grasp the dumbbell with one hand. While rotating the wrist to bring the thumb toward the outside, bend the arm using your biceps. Bring the weight as high as possible. To do this, you may slightly lift the elbow. But do not exaggerate the movement of the elbow (here, the example involves lifting the elbow, but this is only so that you can see the contraction of the biceps).

Maintain the contracted position for one second while squeezing your forearm against your biceps as tightly as possible. Slowly lower the weight to the starting position.

2 3 You can also choose to lift two dumbbells at the same time or one after the other. You will be the strongest if you do this last version.

HELPFUL HINTS
You can either rotate the wrist with every repetition or keep the hand supinated. Use whichever position feels most natural for your arm. If you choose to keep your hand supinated, then do not stretch your arm out completely, especially with heavy weights, because you could tear your biceps muscle. This problem does not occur if you keep the hand neutral when in the outstretched position.

NOTES
With adjustable dumbbells, keep the weights a little off center on the bar. On the side where your pinkie is, place the weights as close as possible to the edge of the bar. This way you will not hit your thigh or torso with the bar.

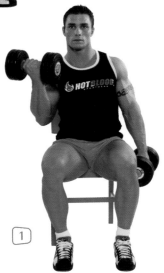

1

(Variations)

1 You can do this exercise while sitting or standing. One possible strategy is to begin the exercise while seated so that you are sure to perform the movement correctly. At failure, stand up so that you can do a few more repetitions by cheating a bit.

ARMS

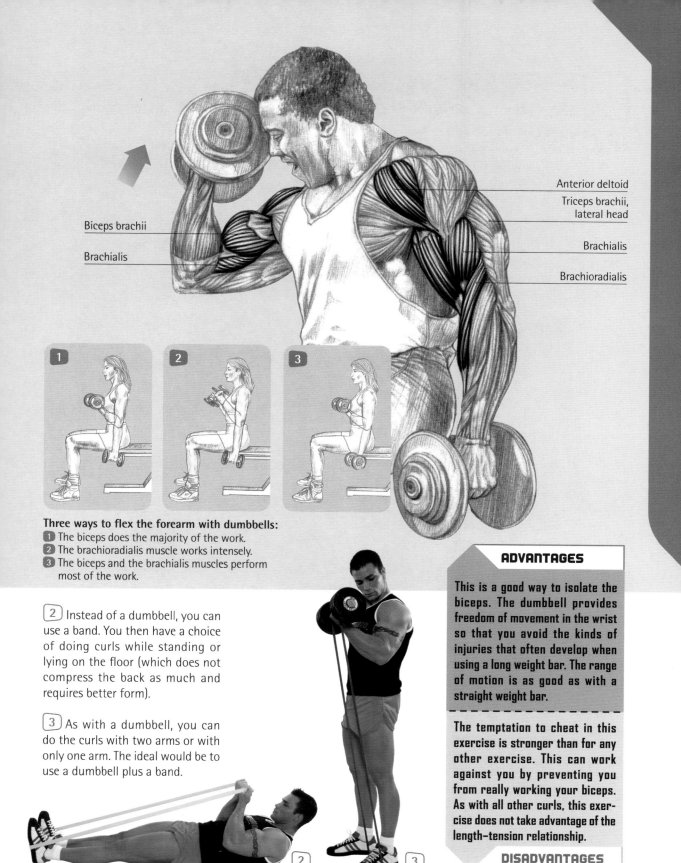

Anterior deltoid

Triceps brachii, lateral head

Brachialis

Brachioradialis

Biceps brachii

Brachialis

Three ways to flex the forearm with dumbbells:
1 The biceps does the majority of the work.
2 The brachioradialis muscle works intensely.
3 The biceps and the brachialis muscles perform
  most of the work.

2 Instead of a dumbbell, you can use a band. You then have a choice of doing curls while standing or lying on the floor (which does not compress the back as much and requires better form).

3 As with a dumbbell, you can do the curls with two arms or with only one arm. The ideal would be to use a dumbbell plus a band.

ADVANTAGES

This is a good way to isolate the biceps. The dumbbell provides freedom of movement in the wrist so that you avoid the kinds of injuries that often develop when using a long weight bar. The range of motion is as good as with a straight weight bar.

The temptation to cheat in this exercise is stronger than for any other exercise. This can work against you by preventing you from really working your biceps. As with all other curls, this exercise does not take advantage of the length-tension relationship.

DISADVANTAGES

/// Hammer Curl

As opposed to supinated curls, **this isolation exercise specifically targets the brachialis and brachioradialis muscles** and does not work the biceps as much. Unilateral work is possible, especially if your primary goal is to have big arms.

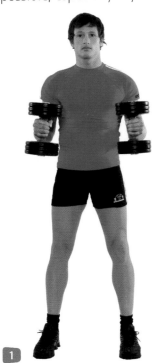

> **!** Be careful of your back and your wrists, especially if you are using very heavy weights.

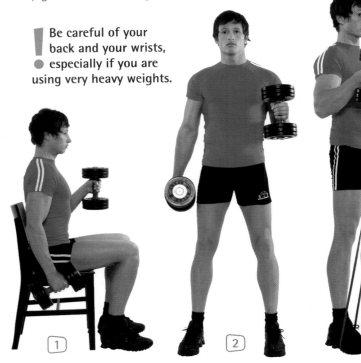

1

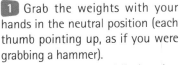

1 Grab the weights with your hands in the neutral position (each thumb pointing up, as if you were grabbing a hammer).

Bend your arms while keeping the thumbs pointing up. Lift the weights as high as possible. To achieve this, you can move the elbows slightly, but be careful not to move them too much. Maintain the contracted position for one second by squeezing your forearms as tightly as possible against your biceps. Lower the weights slowly to the starting position.

COMMENTS
The need to do this exercise will be dictated by the size of your brachialis muscle. If it is the same size as your biceps, then this exercise will not do much for you. If, as is often the case, your brachialis muscle is underdeveloped compared to your biceps, then doing hammer curls makes a lot of sense. Hammer curls can even replace classic (supinated) curls until your brachialis muscle has caught up to your biceps.

Variations

1 You can do this exercise while sitting or standing. One possible strategy is to begin the exercise while seated. At failure, stand up so that you can do a few more repetitions by cheating a bit.

2 You can also choose to lift two dumbbells at the same time or one after the other. You will be the strongest if you do this last version.

3 Instead of a dumbbell, you can use a band or, ideally, a dumbbell plus a band. If you use only a band, you can do the exercise while standing or lying on the floor. In this last version, the back is not compressed as much and the form is better.

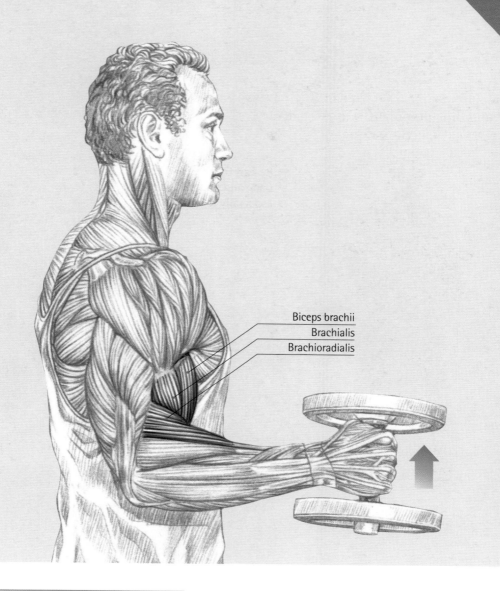

Biceps brachii
Brachialis
Brachioradialis

HELPFUL HINTS

The arm is stronger when you use the neutral hand position than when you use the supinated hand position. So it is normal to be able to use heavier weights with hammer curls than with classic curls. You just have to be careful not to reduce your range of motion because you have picked too heavy a weight.

NOTES

If you are a beginner, you can do either classic curls or hammer curls. However, you should not do both during the same workout. Ideally, you should alternate so that you do classic curls in one workout and hammer curls in the next workout. The relationship between the two will be determined by the development of your biceps and your brachialis muscles, respectively. Another alternative is to do classic curls until you reach failure and then finish in a superset with hammer curls (tapering or not).

ADVANTAGES

The strengthening of the forearm that occurs with hammer curls helps to prevent pain that frequently develops during weight training when the forearms are too weak. As with all curls done unilaterally, you can help yourself with your free hand and do a few forced repetitions.

Hammer curls are not necessarily useful in a weight training program since classic curls and back exercises are already supposed to work the brachialis muscle.

DISADVANTAGES

/// Reverse Curl

This isolation exercise specifically targets the brachioradialis muscle. It also works the brachialis muscle to a lesser extent and a little bit of the biceps. Unilateral work is possible but not essential.

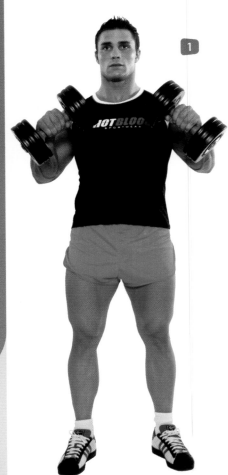

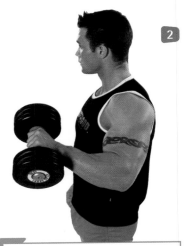

! Be careful of your wrist. Always keep your thumb a little higher than your pinkie finger so you can keep the forearm from twisting too much.

1 Pick up a dumbbell with each hand using a pronated grip (thumbs facing each other). Bend the arms while keeping the thumbs a little higher than your pinkie fingers. Lift the weights as high as possible. Contrary to the other curls, do not lift the elbows during this exercise so that you can really maintain the contraction of the brachioradialis muscles.

2 Maintain the contracted position for one second while squeezing your forearms as tightly as possible against your biceps. Slowly lower the weights to the starting position.

HELPFUL HINTS
The arms are in a relatively weak position, so you must use considerably less weight for reverse curls than for other kinds of curls.

NOTES
You can begin the exercise with reverse curls. At failure, turn the wrists a little and continue the exercise doing hammer curls.

COMMENTS
Whether or not you should do this exercise will be determined by the size of your brachioradialis muscles. If they are well developed from doing other curls, then this exercise will not be especially useful.

ARMS

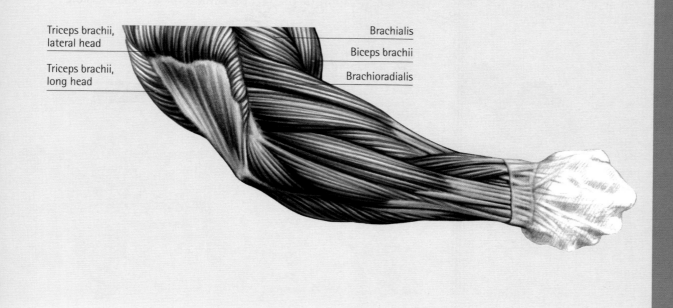

Triceps brachii,
lateral head

Triceps brachii,
long head

Brachialis

Biceps brachii

Brachioradialis

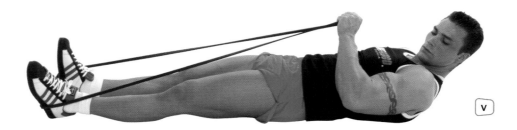

v

Variations

v You can do this exercise while sitting or standing. Begin the exercise while seated. At failure, stand up so that you can do a few more repetitions by cheating a bit.

You can also use a band, which is less traumatic for the wrists than dumbbells. With a band, you can do the exercise while standing or while lying on the floor, unilaterally or bilaterally.

ADVANTAGES

The wrist does not twist as much with dumbbells as it does with a long weight bar. You can prevent injuries by using dumbbells instead of a straight weight bar for this exercise.

In an ideal world, this exercise would be superfluous because, in theory, working the biceps and the back should give you a well-developed brachioradialis muscle.

DISADVANTAGES

/// Concentration Curl

This isolation exercise works the brachialis muscle a bit more and the biceps a bit less than classic (supinated) curls. It particularly emphasizes the interior of the biceps. It is only done unilaterally.

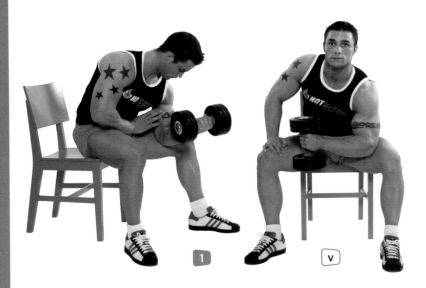

1 While seated, grab a dumbbell with one supinated hand (thumb away from your body). Place your triceps against the inside of your thigh. Bend the arm using your biceps. Lift the weight as high as possible without lifting the elbow. Maintain this contracted position for one second while squeezing your forearm against your biceps as tightly as possible. Slowly lower the weight to the starting position.

(Variations)

v You can use a supinated grip or a hammer grip (thumb pointing up). In the latter version, the brachialis muscle has to work even harder.

HELPFUL HINTS

This exercise is supposed to work the peak of the biceps, giving it a more round form. This is because the brachialis has to work more as well. By pushing the biceps up, the brachialis tends to slightly alter the form of the biceps.

NOTES

Begin your series with concentration curls (supinated or neutral grip); at failure, change to classic curls so you can get a few additional repetitions.

! So that you can be low enough to support your arm on your thigh, you have to round your back. It is therefore vulnerable. To protect your back, press your free hand against your other thigh to create pressure on your spinal column.

ADVANTAGES

By working the brachialis muscle a bit more than classic curls do, concentration curls help to balance the development of the brachialis muscle compared to the biceps muscle.

This exercise is not the most helpful at increasing muscle mass. It is popular mostly because it is relatively easy to do. Since it is done unilaterally, it takes more time.

DISADVANTAGES

ARMS

70

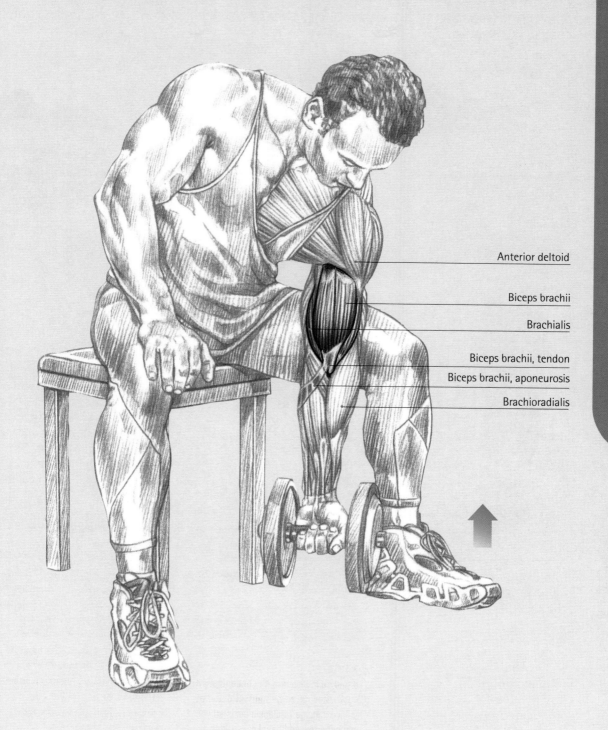

Anterior deltoid

Biceps brachii

Brachialis

Biceps brachii, tendon

Biceps brachii, aponeurosis

Brachioradialis

71

/// Close-Grip Chin-Up

This exercise works not only the biceps but also the back muscles.
It is the only classic multijoint exercise for the biceps. Unilateral work
is next to impossible except for very slight people.

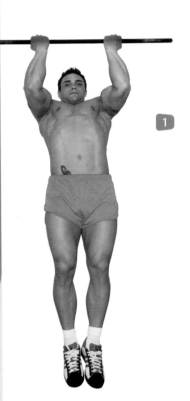

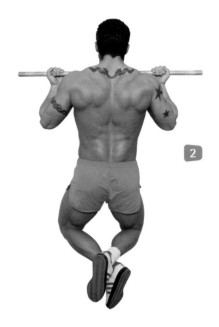

> **HELPFUL HINTS**
> Unlike back exercises in which you try to
> work the biceps as little as possible, here
> the objective is to use the biceps as much as
> possible. You are not trying to contract the
> muscles in the back. To do this exercise, lean
> slightly backward and bring the bar as close to
> your neck as you can.

1 Grab the bar with supinated
hands (pinkie fingers facing each
other). Your hands should be about
shoulder-width apart. If it does not
hurt your wrists, you can move
the hands even closer together.
The closer the grip, the harder the
biceps muscles have to work.

2 Pull yourself up using the
strength of your biceps muscles.
You do not need to touch the bar.
You will reach the height of the
movement when the biceps are well
contracted. Hold the position for
one second before slowly lowering
yourself down.

Variations

v To work the brachioradialis muscle, you can do a pull-up using a
pronated grip (thumbs facing each
other). The biceps will work less,
so you will not be as strong in this
position.

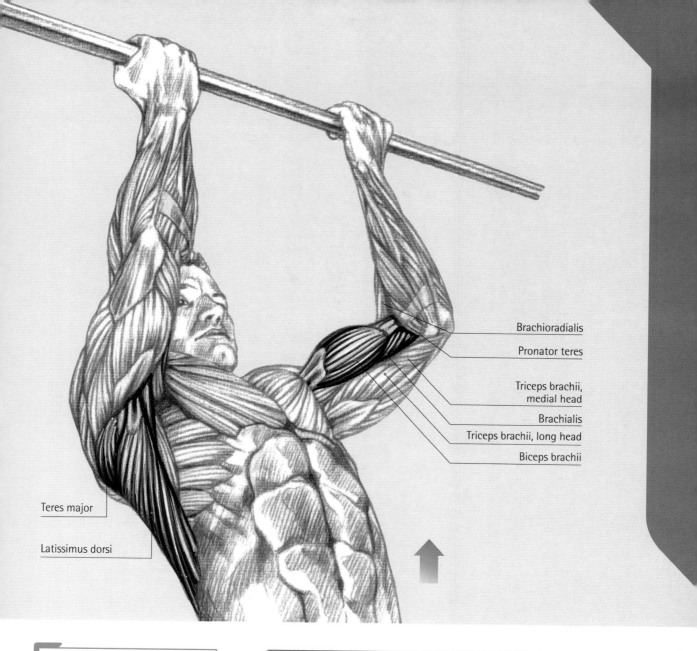

Brachioradialis

Pronator teres

Triceps brachii, medial head

Brachialis

Triceps brachii, long head

Biceps brachii

Teres major

Latissimus dorsi

NOTES

Chin-ups allow you to work the back and the arms simultaneously, which will save time during your workout.

! As with all pulling exercises, do not stretch out the arms completely with supinated hands (pinkie fingers facing each other) since it puts the biceps in a position where they are susceptible to tearing.

ADVANTAGES

Chin-ups are the only classic multijoint exercise for the biceps. They stretch the biceps near the shoulders while contracting them near the elbows. Chin-ups use the length–tension relationship perfectly, which makes them an excellent exercise for quickly gaining arm strength.

Unfortunately, not everyone is capable of doing a chin-up. In this case, you can push your feet off the floor to lighten the load or you can simply do the descending part of the movement (negative part only) and use a chair to help you back up.

DISADVANTAGES

/// Stretch Curl

This is an isolation exercise for the exterior of the biceps since that part of the biceps is responsible for stretching the arm. Since the exterior head of the biceps is the most visible part of the arm, it is the part you should develop first. This exercise can be done only unilaterally.

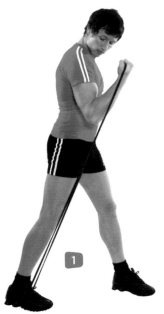

HELPFUL HINTS

Stretching the biceps in this exercise involves a rapid and unique burn. To make the most of this opportunity, do at least 12 repetitions. Once you feel the burn, try to keep it for as long as possible.

NOTES

You can also combine the use of the band with a dumbbell for more effective work.

If you attach the band to a fixed point about midheight, you will get an even bigger stretch out of the biceps.

1 Begin standing with a band under your right foot. Put the right foot behind you and pull on the band with your right arm until you feel considerable resistance. Using your biceps, bring your forearm up to your shoulder while keeping your hand in a supinated position (pinkie toward the body).

Lift the elbow only slightly in order to get the greatest possible contraction. Maintain the contracted position for one second before returning to the starting position. Once you are finished working the right arm, switch to the left arm, taking the shortest possible rest breaks.

! As will all biceps exercises, do not completely straighten the arm while in the lengthened position. In that position, the biceps is susceptible to tearing. Keep good form so that you do not excessively stretch your shoulder.

/// Stretching the Biceps

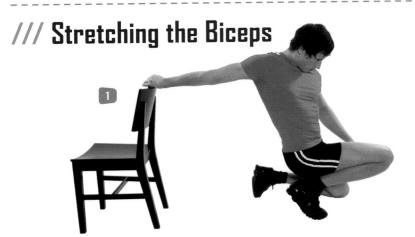

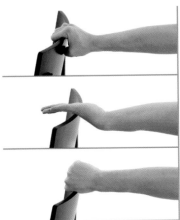

ARMS

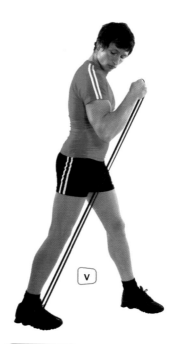

v

Variations

v To work the brachialis muscle a little bit more, you can use the hammer grip (thumb pointing up) instead of the supinated hand position. You can also begin your set with the supinated hand position, and, at failure, rotate your wrist so that your hand is in neutral position. Continue the exercise, moving your foot to release the band a bit so that you decrease the resistance and can do a few more repetitions.

1 To really stretch the biceps, place one hand on the back of a chair. Turn your back very slowly toward the chair. Rotate your wrist from high to low and then low to high so you can really stretch the two heads that form the biceps. Do not make any jerky movements; your muscle is in a very vulnerable position.

Triceps

▌Role of the Triceps

The triceps is the antagonistic muscle to the biceps and the brachialis. It extends the arm, to which it gives much of its mass. Ideally, it should be a little bigger than the biceps and brachialis combined. Unfortunately, it is frequently underdeveloped. But by working it regularly, you can quickly add inches to your arm circumference.

There are three parts to the triceps. The lateral head (on the exterior) is the most visible. The other two heads are somewhat hidden by the torso. Therefore, you should focus on developing the lateral head so you can quickly begin looking like you have very large arms.

! Unexpectedly, the long head of the triceps is involved in all back exercises. Of the three parts of the triceps, it is the only one that is a multijoint muscle. The long head does not just extend the arm. Working together with the back muscles, it is also involved in bringing the arm toward the body. For this reason, you must carefully warm up your elbow before working your back so you can avoid the elbow injuries that are so common.

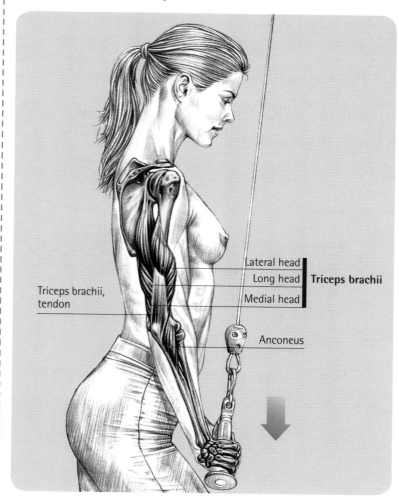

Triceps brachii, tendon

Lateral head
Long head **Triceps brachii**
Medial head

Anconeus

/// Close-Grip Push-Up

This is a multijoint exercise for the triceps, shoulders, and chest. Unilateral work is possible, but only for very light people.

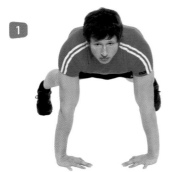

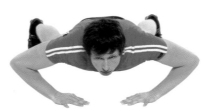

1 Stretch out with your hands on the floor about shoulder-width apart. If you do not have any pain in your wrists, then you can move your hands closer together.

2 Lower yourself slowly. Once on the floor, raise yourself using your triceps as much as possible.

HELPFUL HINTS
To better work the exterior of the triceps, turn your hands slightly toward each other. Another possibility is to vary the angle between the torso and the arms. Find the position where you feel the triceps the most, somewhere between having your hands in line with the shoulders and having them in line with the chest.

NOTES
The closer your grip, the more you will feel the triceps. However, if you are using your chest muscles even a little bit, then you will be weaker when you use a close grip.

Variations

To add resistance, wrap a band around your back and hold it in both of your hands.

1 Loop the band only once around your back when you begin.

2 When you are stronger, you can put both loops around your back.

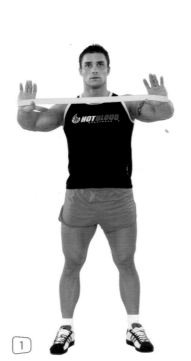

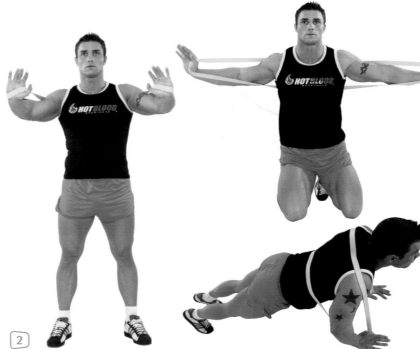

1

2

ARMS

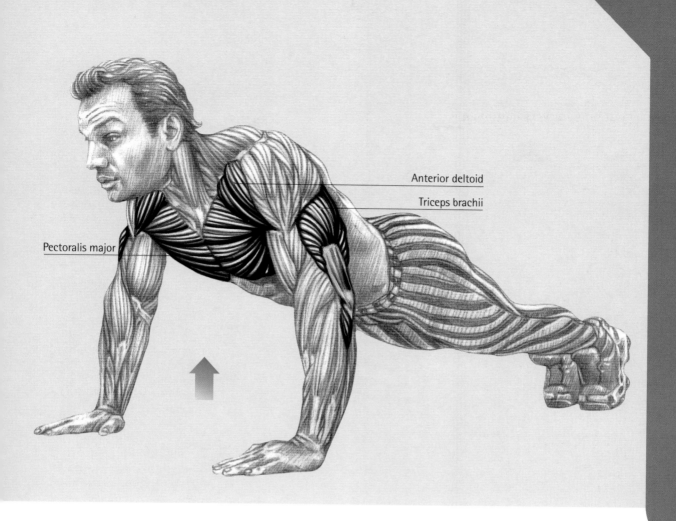

Anterior deltoid

Triceps brachii

Pectoralis major

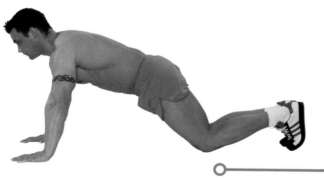

Not all wrists are made for push-ups. To avoid injuring them, you can use dumbbells on the floor, which make gripping easier. Special push-up bars are also available in sporting goods stores. They increase the range of motion during the exercise while preventing too much unnatural tension in the wrists.

ADVANTAGES

It is easy to vary the resistance. If your body is too heavy, begin doing push-ups on your knees rather than on your feet so that you can gain strength. In the same way, at the end of a set in which you are doing push-ups from the feet, if you are not strong enough to do any more regular push-ups, then go to your knees and do a few more repetitions. Push-ups are one of the only exercises for the triceps that take advantage of the length-tension relationship of the long head.

- -

It is not easy to focus your work on the triceps. In addition, push-ups do not always work well for every person's anatomy. If you have long arms, then it will be more difficult with no guarantee of good results.

DISADVANTAGES

/// Triceps Extension, Seated or Standing, With Dumbbell

This is an isolation exercise for the triceps.
It can be done unilaterally.

! When doing this exercise bilaterally, it is easy to lose your form, arch your back, or hit yourself in the head with a weight.

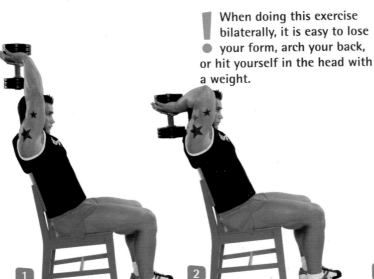

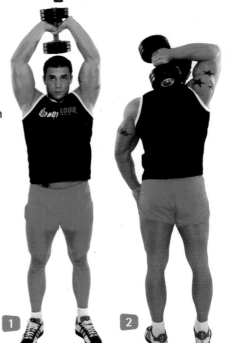

1 Sit or stand. Grab a dumbbell with both hands (for bilateral work) or with one hand (for unilateral work).

2 Move the weight behind your head, with your elbows and pinkie fingers pointing toward the ceiling. Using your triceps, straighten your arms before bringing the weight back down.

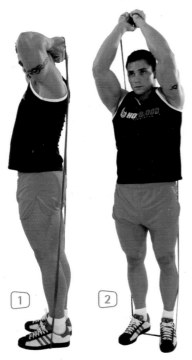

HELPFUL HINTS
The range of motion is much greater when this exercise is done unilaterally because the stretch is better and the contraction is more pronounced.

NOTES
Do not confuse this exercise with a pullover exercise. At all times, the arms remain more or less perpendicular to the floor.

Variations

1 You can also do this exercise with a band. Hold one end in your hands and put the other end under your feet. Using a band, you can change from a pronated to a neutral to a supinated grip.

2 If you are working bilaterally, it is best to maintain continuous tension. This means that you never completely stretch out your arms. However, if you are working unilaterally, you can stretch the arm so that you get a really good triceps contraction.

ADVANTAGES

This exercise provides a good stretch, which is rather unique among triceps exercises.

The elbows are really worked during this exercise. You must control the movement to avoid hurting the elbow joint. This movement does not really make use of the length-tension relationship in the triceps.

DISADVANTAGES

ARMS

78

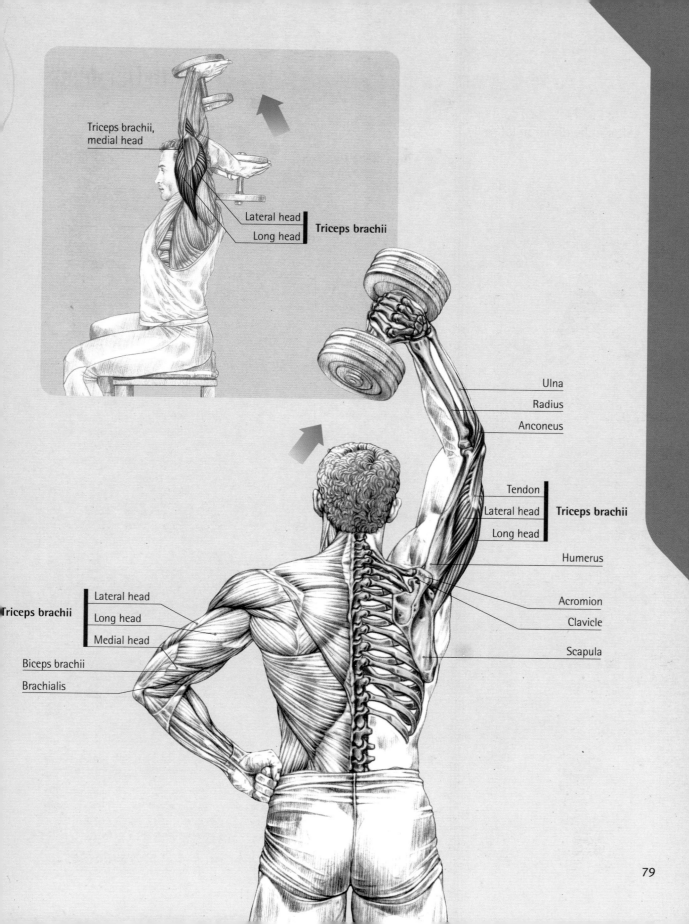

Triceps brachii, medial head

Lateral head

Long head

Triceps brachii

Ulna

Radius

Anconeus

Tendon

Lateral head

Long head

Triceps brachii

Humerus

Acromion

Clavicle

Scapula

Triceps brachii

Lateral head

Long head

Medial head

Biceps brachii

Brachialis

79

/// Lying Triceps Extension

This is an isolation exercise for the triceps. It can be done unilaterally.

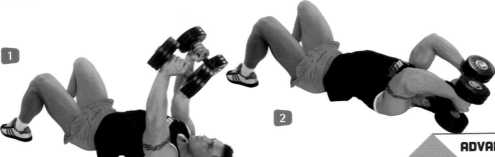

1 Lie on your back on the floor and grab the dumbbells.

> ⚠ **Be careful not to hit your head with the dumbbell, especially when you get tired and your form deteriorates.**

2 Lower the weights behind your head with hands in neutral position (pinkie fingers toward the ceiling). Stretch the triceps to their maximum without moving the arms too much. Elbows should remain pointed toward the ceiling. Using your triceps, lift the weights. Contract for one second before you lower the weights.

ADVANTAGES

The back is well protected when you are lying down. Your form will be better than when you do the extensions while standing up.

- - - - - - - - - - - - - - - - -

The elbows are worked hard during this exercise. You must perform the movement with great control so that you do not injure the elbows. The length-tension relationship of the triceps is not used as much as it should be for optimal effectiveness.

DISADVANTAGES

HELPFUL HINTS
It is possible to start with the dumbbell behind your head or by your ears. Choose your starting point depending on what feels most natural for your elbows.

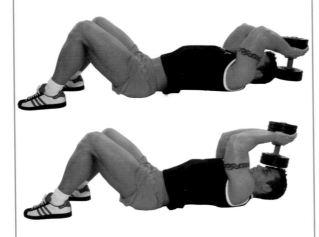

NOTES
Do not confuse this exercise with a pullover exercise. At all times, the arms remain more or less perpendicular to the floor.

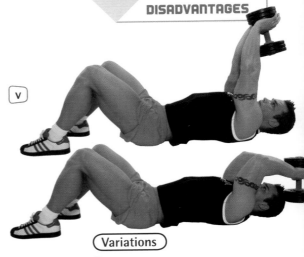

Variations

V Even if you are working bilaterally, you can use one or two dumbbells. To learn the proper form, you should begin with just one dumbbell and hold it with both of your hands, as in the previous exercise. In this way, you will be able to control the weight better.

ARMS

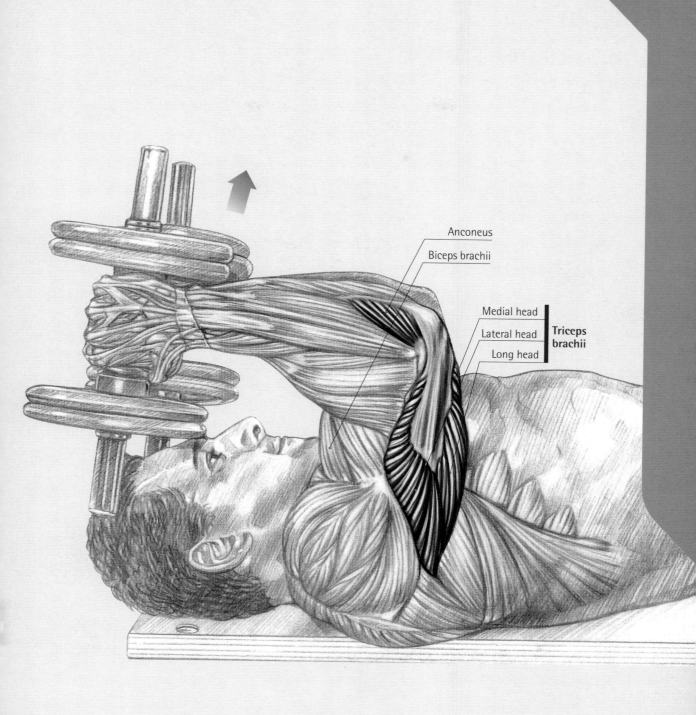

Anconeus

Biceps brachii

Medial head

Lateral head **Triceps brachii**

Long head

81

/// Triceps Kickback

This is an isolation exercise for the triceps; you can do it unilaterally.

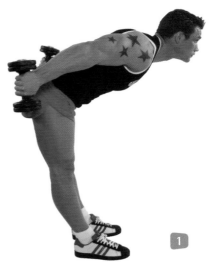

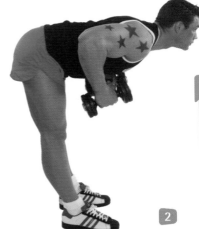

1 While leaning forward, grab the dumbbells with your hands in the neutral position (thumbs pointing toward the floor). Your arms should be glued to your sides and parallel to the floor.

2 Lower the weights so that your forearms are perpendicular to the floor. Using your triceps, straighten your arms. Hold the position for one second with arms extended before lowering the weights.

HELPFUL HINTS
When your arms are extended, hold the position for as long as you can so that you contract the triceps as much as possible. In fact, unlike regular triceps exercises, you have to generate a lot of muscular tension in order to keep your arms extended during this exercise. Take full advantage of this unique feature.

NOTES
By turning your pinkie finger slightly to the outside in the contracted position, you can focus the work on the exterior of the triceps.

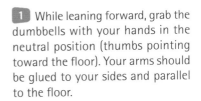

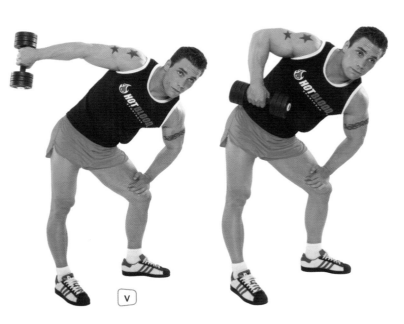

(**Variations**)

v You can either keep the elbow toward the back or lift it a little toward the ceiling. This latter version helps some people to feel the work of the triceps a little better. It is better to do this version unilaterally so that you have more stability.

! The lower back is involved when you do this exercise bilaterally.
● When you do the exercise unilaterally, you can press your free hand against the thigh, which will help support the spinal column.

ARMS

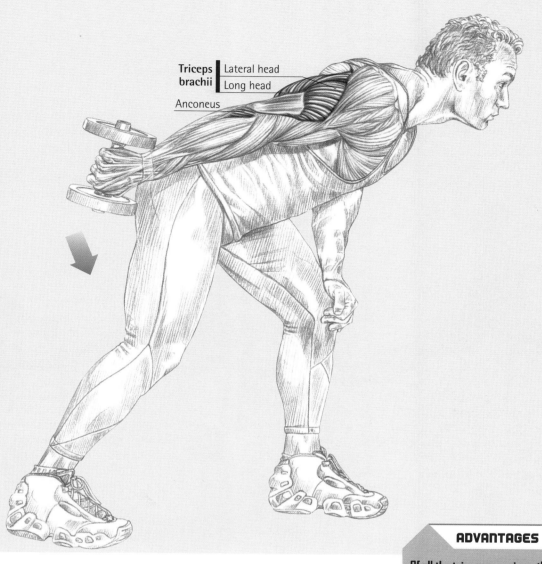

Triceps brachii — Lateral head / Long head

Anconeus

/// Reverse Dip

This is a multijoint exercise for the triceps, chest, and shoulders.
This exercise cannot be done unilaterally.

HELPFUL HINTS
When you lift yourself up using your triceps muscles, keep your head straight and your eyes looking slightly toward the ceiling.

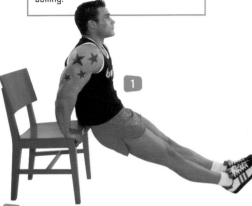

1 Turn your back to a chair or your bed and place your hands on the edge with pronated wrists (thumbs facing each other). Keep your legs straight out in front of you.

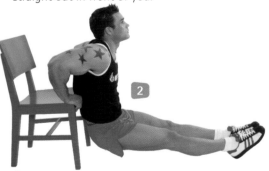

2 Bend your arms to lower your body toward the floor, and then use your triceps to lift yourself back up. You do not need to have a very large range of motion; about 18 inches (45 cm) should suffice.

! Be careful to maintain stability, especially if your feet are elevated. If you lose your grip, you could hurt yourself.

NOTES
When this exercise becomes too easy, put a chair in front of you so that you can put your feet on it. In this way, your triceps will have to move more of your body weight. One possible combination is to begin with your feet on a chair and then, at failure, finish the exercise with your feet on the floor to get the maximum number of repetitions.

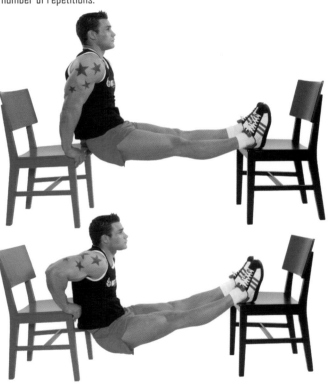

To increase resistance even more, place a weight on your upper thighs.

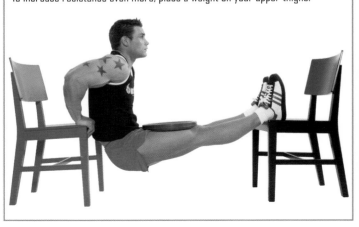

ARMS

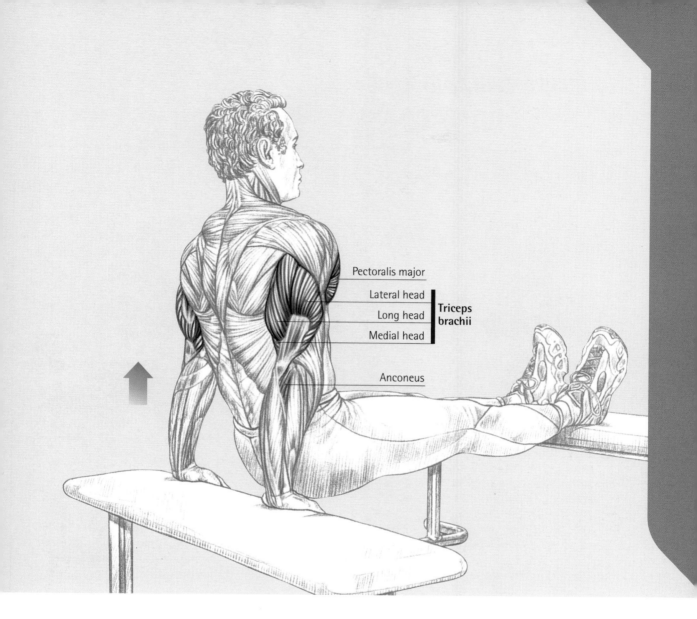

Pectoralis major

Lateral head

Long head   Triceps
              brachii

Medial head

Anconeus

Variations

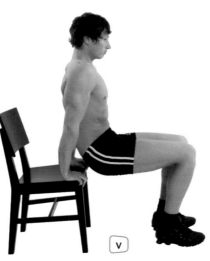

[v] Vary the width of your hands until you find the position where your triceps muscles work the most. If you keep your legs bent, then the exercise is much easier. One possible combination for a beginner is to begin with straight legs, and then at failure, bend the legs in order to get a few more repetitions.

[v]

/// Push-Down With a Band

This is an isolation exercise for the triceps. It can be done unilaterally.

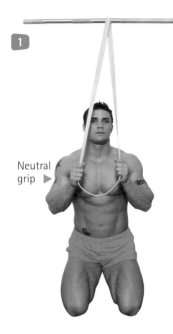

1 Neutral grip ▶

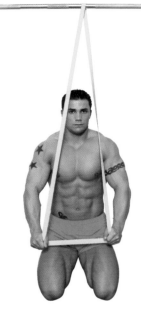

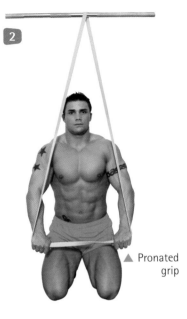

2

▲ Pronated grip

1 Attach a band to your pull-up bar. If you do not have a pull-up bar, then attach one end of the band to the top of a door. Get on your knees with your arms at 90 degrees, and grab the band with your hands in neutral position (thumbs pointing up) or in pronated position (thumbs facing each other). You can also use an intermediate grip somewhere between pronated and neutral. Use whichever grip allows you to contract the triceps the most.

2 Pull on the band so that you stretch your arms. Hold the position for one second before returning to the starting position.

ADVANTAGES

Working with a band is less traumatic for the elbow joint than body-weight or dumbbell exercises.

- - - - - - - - - - - - - - - - -

It is difficult to measure the exact resistance with a band alone. The length-tension relationship is not used to the most benefit when you do the exercise with the band in front of you. It is a little better in the version just described.

DISADVANTAGES

Variations

v If the band is attached to a pull-up bar, you can turn your back to it. Lean forward with the biceps going away from your head. This is a better stretch for the triceps.

HELPFUL HINTS
At first, it is better to do this exercise slowly so that you can really feel the triceps. In fact, since the triceps is not used on a daily basis, many beginners have trouble feeling this muscle.

NOTES
You can vary the width of your hands in the contracted position. You should not be constantly changing the position of your hands, though. Simply find the position that works best for you, because it is rare that all grips are equally efficient.

ARMS

/// Plyometric Exercises for the Triceps

1 The main plyometric exercise for the triceps is push-ups against the wall or on the floor. Begin the standing version against a wall so that you can get used to the exercise. When you stand facing a wall, your hands should be about shoulder-width apart.

2 Let yourself fall against the wall. At the last moment, use your arms to push off the wall so that you do not hit it.

  The farther you move away from the wall, the harder the exercise will be.

ADVANTAGES

This exercise will make you stronger in all exercises where you need to push against an opponent or an object, such as rugby, martial arts, and shot put.

Do not overestimate your strength and end up hitting your head on the floor.

DISADVANTAGES

! This exercise seriously works the elbow and shoulder joints.

Variations

Once you are comfortable standing up close to the wall, move farther away from the wall. When you feel ready, then you can change to the floor version. At first, do the exercise on your knees, and then move to the regular version.

/// Stretching the Triceps

1 Lift your right arm so that your biceps is right next to your head. Hold a band in your right hand and pull on it with your left hand so that your right arm bends as much as possible. Ideally, your right hand would touch your right shoulder.

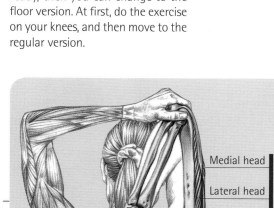

Medial head
Lateral head — Triceps brachii
Long head

Forearms

Role of the Forearms

Many of the muscles of the forearm are multijoint, so they are simultaneously involved in these actions:

> Moving the hand by closing and opening it
> Moving the wrist by raising and lowering the hand
> Moving the elbow by raising and lowering the forearm

The forearm muscles are involved in all weight training movements of the arm and torso (except for the abdominals). Their strength can be a limiting factor in many exercises. If they are weak, you will need to strengthen them. Even though powerful forearms are omnipresent in the gym, they are not useful in many sports. So you will have to decide how much to work them depending on your needs while keeping in mind that direct work is not strictly necessary.

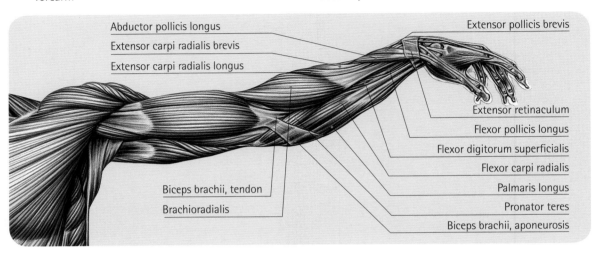

- Abductor pollicis longus
- Extensor carpi radialis brevis
- Extensor carpi radialis longus
- Extensor pollicis brevis
- Extensor retinaculum
- Flexor pollicis longus
- Flexor digitorum superficialis
- Flexor carpi radialis
- Palmaris longus
- Pronator teres
- Biceps brachii, aponeurosis
- Biceps brachii, tendon
- Brachioradialis

/// Wrist Curl

This is an isolation exercise for the internal part of the forearm. Unilateral work is possible, but not necessarily desirable since you do not want to lose too much time during a workout.

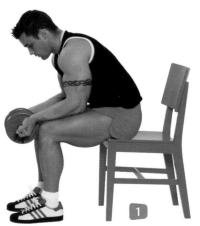

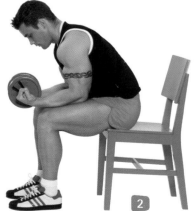

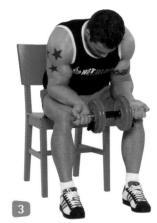

1 While seated, grab the dumbbell at the ends with supinated hands (thumbs toward the outside). Put the forearms on the thighs so that your hands can move freely.

2 Using your forearms, lift the weight as high as possible. Hold the contraction for one second before slowly lowering the weight.

3 The more you bend your arms, the stronger you will be during this exercise.

ARMS

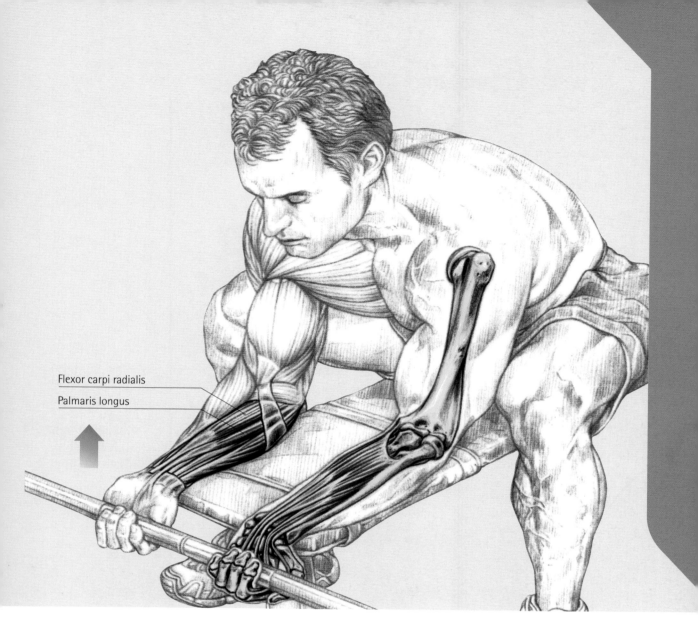

Flexor carpi radialis

Palmaris longus

! The wrists are fragile and yet very heavily used
joints. This is why it is better to do more repetitions
● (15 to 25) with a lighter weight rather than fewer
repetitions with a very heavy weight.

Variations

Unilateral work is possible but
more dangerous because doing
this makes the wrist more flexible.
When stretched, the wrist is in a
somewhat precarious position. Do
not push too hard at the lower end
of the range of motion during this
exercise.

ADVANTAGES

Wrist curls can allow you more
strength for working the biceps and
the back.

- - - - - - - - - - - - - - - - -

Wrist curls can do double the work in
biceps and back exercises.

DISADVANTAGES

HELPFUL HINTS

This is not a power exercise done
explosively. The muscles in the forearm
were made to sustain prolonged effort.
Do the exercise slowly.

NOTES

The wrist curl is not necessarily a
useful exercise. It is superfluous for
many beginners unless their particular
sports require powerful forearms or
they have really weak forearms.

89

/// Wrist Extension

This is an isolation exercise for the external part of the forearm. The exercise can be done unilaterally, but this is not necessarily the best way to do it.

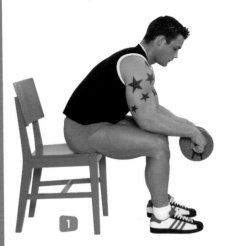

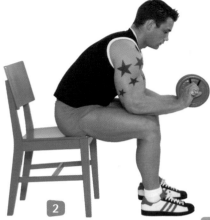

1 Sit down and grab a dumbbell with your hands at the ends. Use a pronated grip (thumbs facing each other). Rest your forearms on your thighs so that your hands can move freely.

2 Using your forearms, lift the weight as high as possible. Hold the contracted position for one second before slowly lowering the weight.

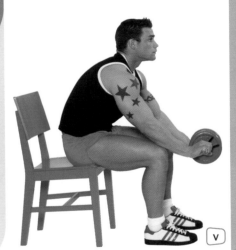

Variations

v Begin the exercise with arms bent at about 90 degrees. At failure, straighten the arms so that you can do a few more repetitions. The straighter your arms, the stronger you will be.

ADVANTAGES

Exercises for the biceps, triceps, and back muscles require a lot of work from the flexor muscles in the wrist (the muscles used for wrist curls). However, the extensor muscles (those that work during wrist extensions) are used to a much lesser degree. You can create an imbalance between the flexors and the extensors, and an injury can result from an imbalance between the antagonistic muscles. Wrist extensions are a more useful exercise than wrist curls because they help balance the development of the wrist muscles.

Wrist curls can still cost you some time and energy if you are a beginner. The work is repeated with reverse curls.

DISADVANTAGES

HELPFUL HINTS

Place your hands on the bar as naturally as possible. If you feel any pulling in your wrists, grab the weight a little lopsided by moving your thumbs slightly toward your body rather than having them directly face each other.

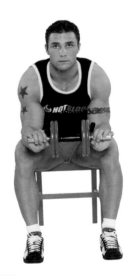

NOTES

A preexhaustion superset can save you time. Begin with wrist curls and, at failure, stand up and immediately begin doing reverse curls so that you really tire out the muscles.

ARMS

90

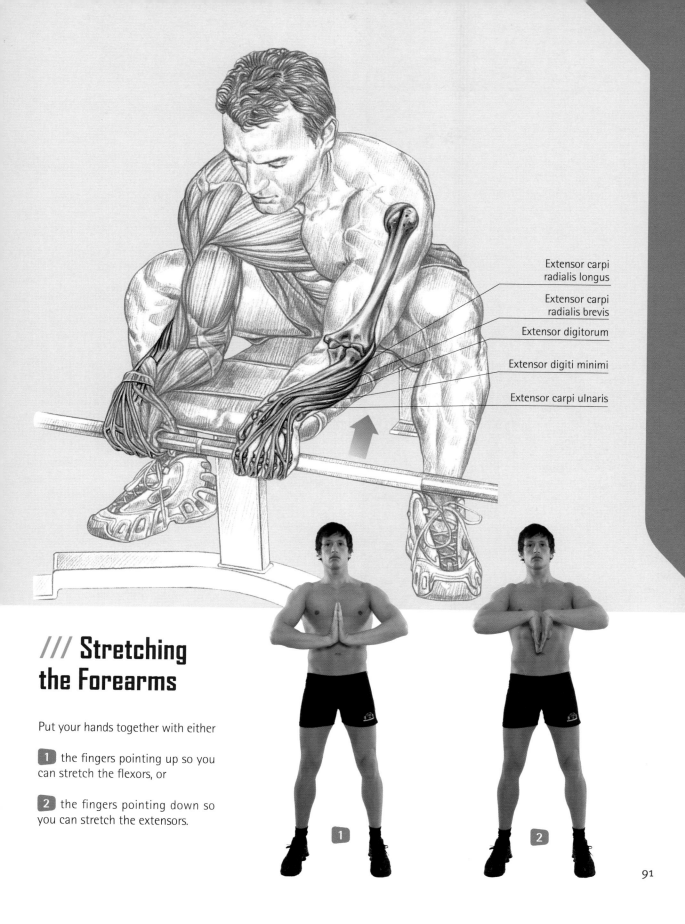

Extensor carpi radialis longus

Extensor carpi radialis brevis

Extensor digitorum

Extensor digiti minimi

Extensor carpi ulnaris

/// Stretching the Forearms

Put your hands together with either

1 the fingers pointing up so you can stretch the flexors, or

2 the fingers pointing down so you can stretch the extensors.

91

DEVELOP BIGGER SHOULDERS

▌Role of the Deltoid

The deltoid is a single-joint muscle that is responsible for arm movement in all directions. Aesthetically, the shoulders define your build. Because of this, it is important to develop them.

In a somewhat artificial manner, the deltoid is divided into three parts:

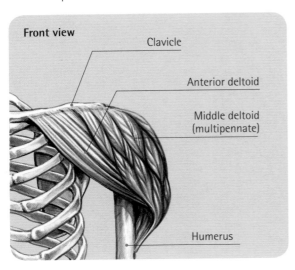

Front view

Clavicle

Anterior deltoid

Middle deltoid (multipennate)

Humerus

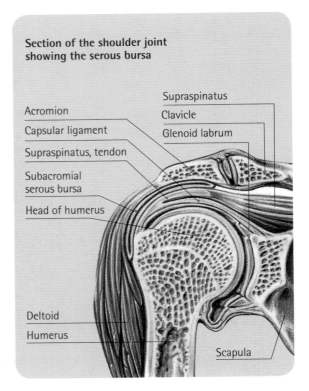

Section of the shoulder joint showing the serous bursa

Supraspinatus

Acromion

Clavicle

Capsular ligament

Glenoid labrum

Supraspinatus, tendon

Subacromial serous bursa

Head of humerus

Deltoid

Humerus

Scapula

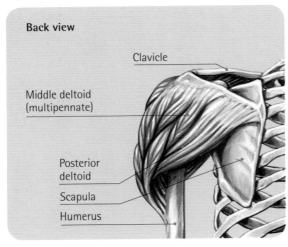

Back view

Clavicle

Middle deltoid (multipennate)

Posterior deltoid

Scapula

Humerus

1. Front of the shoulder. This part lifts the arm in front. The anterior part also works in conjunction with the chest muscles. If you are seriously working your chest, then it may not be useful to focus on the front of the shoulder, especially since this particular zone of the deltoid is the easiest to develop. If you do not specifically work the front of the shoulder in addition to the chest, it will save you time and lighten the burden on your shoulder as well as your elbow.

2. Lateral part of the shoulder. This section raises the arm to the side. This gesture is not very common in sports or in daily life. The role of the middle of the shoulder is mostly aesthetic given its curve and its size in relation to the torso. This is why the lateral part of the deltoid is highly valued.

3. Back of the shoulder. This part pulls the arm backward. It is the most neglected and most underdeveloped part of the shoulder. There is an imbalance between the front of the shoulder (overtrained) and the back of the shoulder (undertrained). Scientific studies have measured this imbalance. Compared to sedentary people, athletes with a good level of fitness have the following features:

> An average of 250 percent greater muscle mass on the front of the shoulder

> 150 percent greater muscle mass on the lateral part of the shoulder

> Only 10 to 15 percent greater muscle mass on the back of the shoulder

Pulled forward by a strong front deltoid and not counterbalanced by a sufficiently powerful back of the shoulder, the shoulder joint moves forward. This creates a hunchback appearance. Aside from aesthetics, the shoulder joint is no longer where it should be, and this opens the door to several problems.

In this book, we try to prevent this very common imbalance in the following ways:

> By cautioning against excessive work on the front of the shoulder
> By highlighting the importance of developing the back of the shoulder

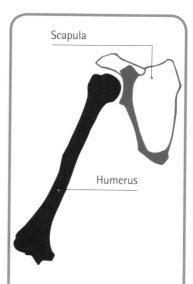

Scapula

Humerus

! Because of the wide range of motion of the arm, the shoulder joint is relatively unstable and therefore fragile. It is the site of numerous injuries and a limiting factor that you must consider in all shoulder exercises. This is even truer since chest, back, and arm exercises involve the shoulder.

/// Dumbbell Press

This is a multijoint exercise for the front of the deltoid, the triceps, and the upper chest. Unilateral work is possible.

Neutral grip ▶

1 While sitting or standing, bring the dumbbells to the height of your head. Use whatever hand position feels most natural for you. In general, the thumb points more or less at your head, but you could also turn it toward the back or the outside.

2 From there, push the weights up and bring them together. Do not completely straighten the arms. Then bring the weights back to the starting position.

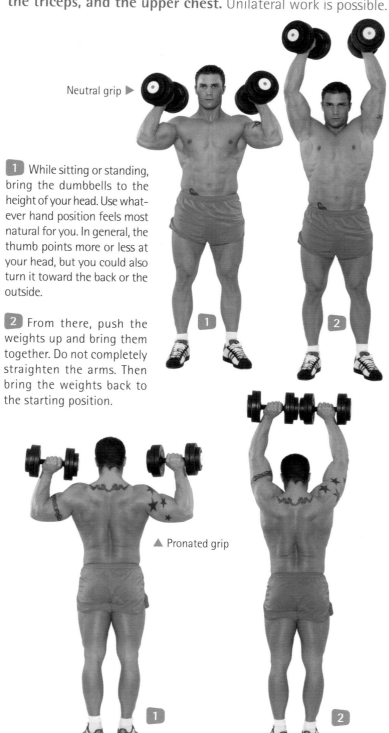

▲ Pronated grip

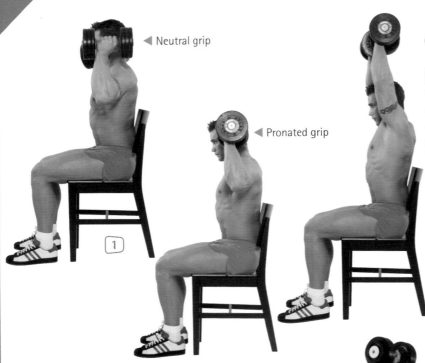

◀ Neutral grip

◀ Pronated grip

(Variations)

1 You can perform this exercise while sitting or standing. If you are bodybuilding to improve your appearance, then it is better to sit down for this exercise so that you are more stable. But in many sports (contact sports in particular), the shoulders and arms must be accustomed to working at the same time as the thighs. In this case, you should do shoulder exercises while standing so that you train your upper-body muscles to work in conjunction with your lower-body muscles.

◀ Alternating unilateral exercise

◀ Simple unilateral exercise

! When your arms are holding a weight above your head, you are in a vulnerable position. If the weight moves your arms backward, you could suffer a serious injury. Be sure that you remain stable and control the weight at all times.

There is a natural tendency to arch the back during this exercise, especially in the standing position. Moving your body backward allows you to do a part of this exercise with the upper-chest muscles. Your strength will be increased, but the shoulders will work less, and you risk hurting your back.

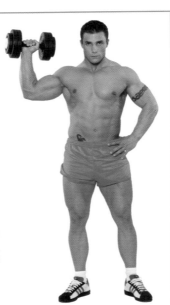

HELPFUL HINTS

You do not have to lower the weight all the way down. Many people prefer to stop the movement when the weight is at the ear. After this point, you could start shaking in the shoulder joint. How far you lower the weight will depend on your flexibility as well as the size of your clavicle. If these two things are not well developed, then you should not lower the weight very far.

NOTES

With most adjustable weights, you can move the weights on the bar so that you do not end up bumping your head. To do this, move the weights as close to the inside of the bar as possible.

2 In sports like the shot put, unilateral work is better. In all other cases, it is better to work bilaterally.

SHOULDERS

Numerous muscles have to work during this one exercise, especially if you do the exercise while standing.

Unless you are weak in the shoulder, then exercises for the front of the shoulder are not always required, especially if you are working the chest a lot. In this case, it is better to focus on the lateral and back parts of the deltoid rather than on the front.

DISADVANTAGES

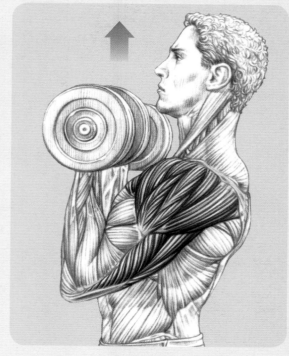

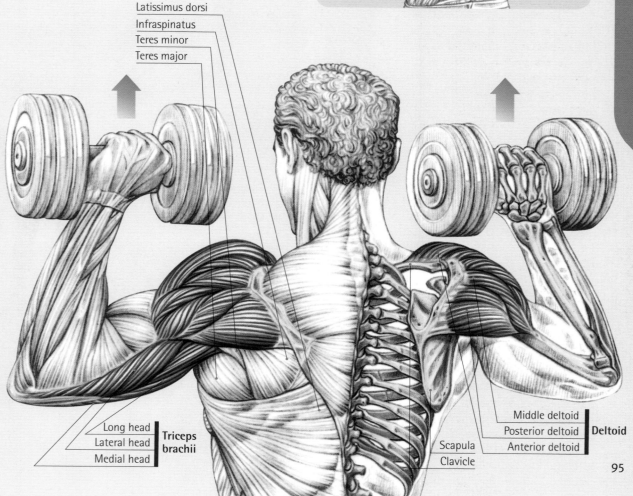

Latissimus dorsi
Infraspinatus
Teres minor
Teres major

Long head
Lateral head   **Triceps brachii**
Medial head

Middle deltoid
Posterior deltoid   **Deltoid**
Anterior deltoid

Scapula
Clavicle

/// Front Lateral Raise

This is an isolation exercise for the front of the deltoid and the upper chest. It can be done unilaterally.

1 Stand with one or two dumbbells in your hands. You can use the classic pronated grip (thumbs facing each other) or a neutral grip (thumbs pointing up). Choose whatever position feels best for you.

2 Using your shoulders, lift the arms at least to your eye level.

3 If you feel comfortable with this, you can lift your arms a little higher (just above the head). The higher you lift your arms, the lighter the weights you will need to use. The sensation of the muscles contracting should guide you in determining the arm height that is best for you; realize that there is no definitive rule for this.

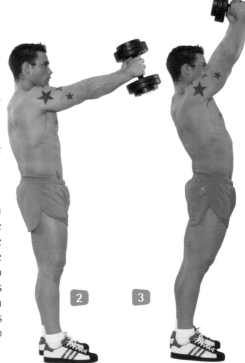

HELPFUL HINTS

It is easy to get carried away and start moving your torso back and forth. It is still better to maintain good form so that you isolate the movement to the front of the shoulder. To avoid cheating, you can do this exercise with your back against a wall.

NOTES

As with all isolation exercises for the shoulder, tapering sets is particularly appropriate. For example, you can begin with two dumbbells and then, at failure, switch to only one dumbbell.

! So that you can use heavier weights, there is a tendency to arch the back. It is better to lean very slightly forward while keeping the back very straight. You will certainly be able to lift heavier weights, but the isolation will be better and there will be less risk of injury.

Variations

1 You can lift both arms at the same time or you can alternate the left and right arms for each repetition. This latter version means you can use heavier weights. You can also use just one dumbbell, holding it with both hands using a neutral grip (thumbs pointing up). This version is undoubtedly better for beginners since it is easier to master at first.

2 You can also use a band by itself or combined with a dumbbell. Use the different hand positions that we have described.

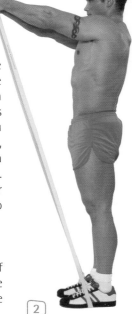

ADVANTAGES

The front of the shoulder is well isolated without interference from the triceps, whose strength can limit the work done by the deltoid in press exercises.

If you do the bench press (or push-ups) for the chest plus shoulder presses, then you do not need to add front lateral raises to your program. However, if you cannot do shoulder presses because of pain in your elbows, then do this exercise instead of the multijoint exercises.

DISADVANTAGES

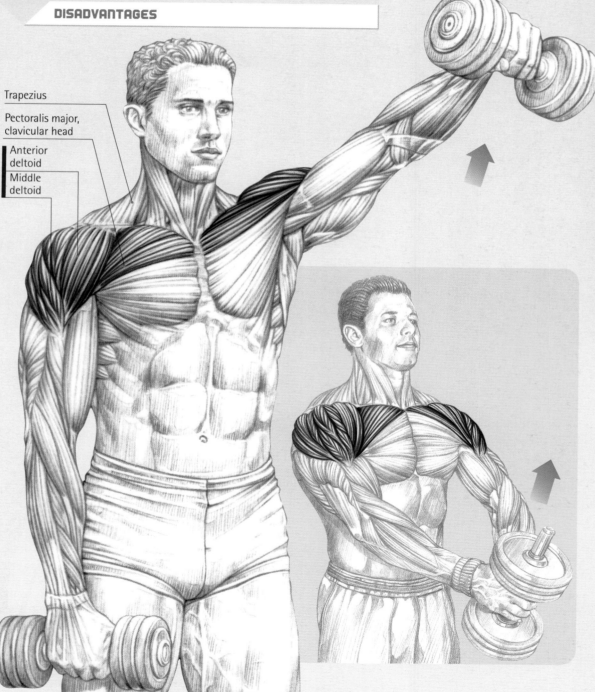

Trapezius

Pectoralis major, clavicular head

Anterior deltoid

Middle deltoid

Deltoid

/// Upright Row

This multijoint exercise works the front as well as the outside of the deltoid.
The biceps and the trapezius muscles are also used. The exercise can be done unilaterally, but this may not be the best way to do it.

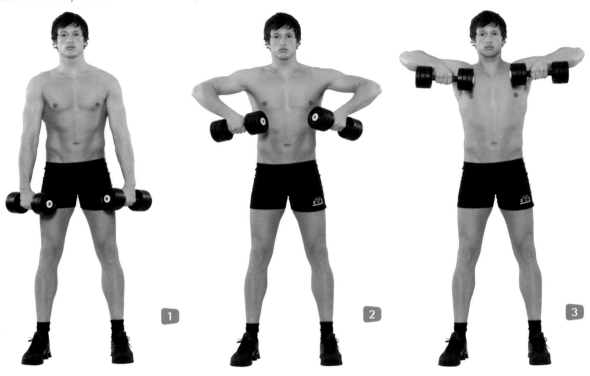

1 Stand with dumbbells in hand, using a pronated grip (thumbs turned toward each other).

2 3 Lift your arms while bending them. Be sure that your weights stay as close to your body as possible at all times.

! To reduce twisting in the wrists, let the dumbbells move as they will. However, you should avoid this exercise if it feels uncomfortable to you.

HELPFUL HINTS
You do not have to lift the weights all the way to your head. Many people prefer to lift the dumbbells only as high as the chest.

NOTES
You can move the hands closer together or farther away. The farther apart they are, the harder the deltoids will work. When the hands are closer together, the trapezius muscles do more of the work.

ADVANTAGES

This is the only multijoint exercise for the shoulders that does not depend on the triceps. If you feel that your triceps limit your strength during shoulder exercises, then you can use upright rows to your advantage. One possible superset would be to combine shoulder presses with upright rows (in this order or in the opposite order, as you wish).

Not everyone can do this exercise without causing injury. In some people, certain parts of the shoulder and wrist joints cannot tolerate this exercise at all. If this is the case for you, then skip this exercise.

DISADVANTAGES

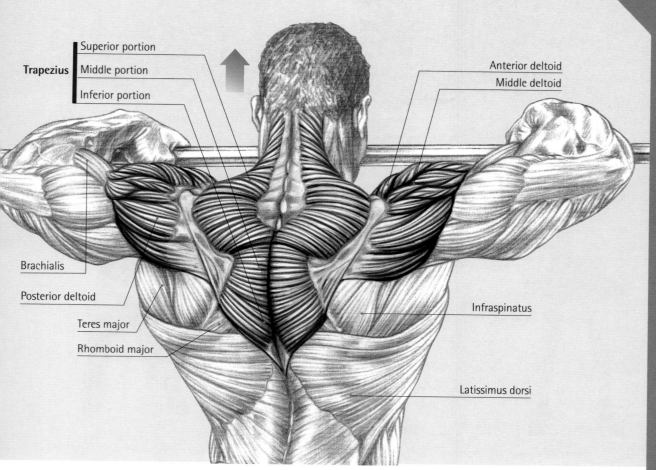

Trapezius
Superior portion
Middle portion
Inferior portion

Anterior deltoid
Middle deltoid

Brachialis

Posterior deltoid

Teres major

Rhomboid major

Infraspinatus

Latissimus dorsi

Variations

1 Instead of dumbbells, you can use a band under your feet. Ideally, you would combine dumbbells and a band.

2 With the band alone, you can do the exercise while lying on the floor, which has the added advantage of reducing pressure on the spinal column.

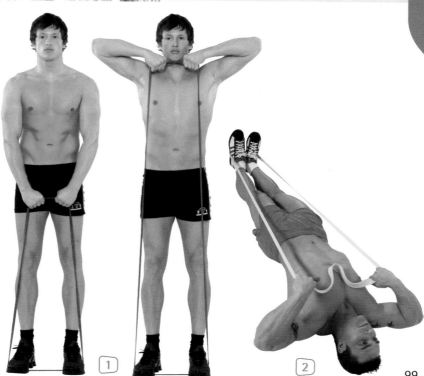

1

2

99

/// Lateral Raise

This is an exercise especially for the lateral part of the shoulder. This is the best isolation exercise for defining your figure.

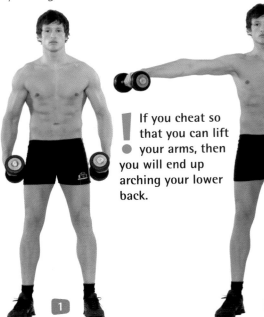

! If you cheat so that you can lift your arms, then you will end up arching your lower back.

1 If you feel good doing this exercise, then you might as well do both arms at the same time. Grab your dumbbells or your band using a neutral grip (thumbs facing forward). Place your hands near the outsides of your thighs.

2 Lift your arms as straight as you possibly can while keeping them in line with your body. Bending the arms makes the exercise easier, but it will not improve the size of your shoulders. At all times during the exercise, the thumbs should be lower than the pinkie fingers so that you really focus your efforts on the lateral part of the deltoids.

TIP
When your shoulders are on fire, holding your arms along your sides between sets will prolong the burn. To drain the lactic acid from the shoulders more quickly, simply hang from a pull-up bar. Gravity will help cleanse the shoulder of metabolic waste. You can also combine lateral raises with chin-ups for the back. This superset of antagonistic muscles is beneficial because it helps the deltoids recover.

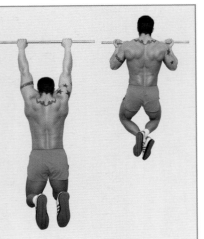

HELPFUL HINTS
You can do this exercise while sitting or standing. In general, form is better when sitting down than when standing. One possible combination is to begin this exercise sitting down, and at failure, stand up so that you can do a few more repetitions using a little bit of momentum.

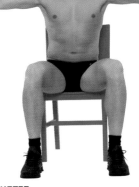

NOTES
On at least the first few repetitions, you should be able to stop completely with your arms parallel to the floor. If you cannot stop cleanly, it means you are using too much momentum to complete the movement and your weight is too heavy.

ADVANTAGES

Since the isolation of the deltoids is almost perfect, you can easily do tapering sets to work the muscles deeply. You will not have any interference from the triceps or any other muscle wearing out before the deltoids.

To defy gravity, there is a strong tendency to cheat in this exercise, which is counterproductive. Since this is an isolation exercise, you will not be able to use very heavy weights.

DISADVANTAGES

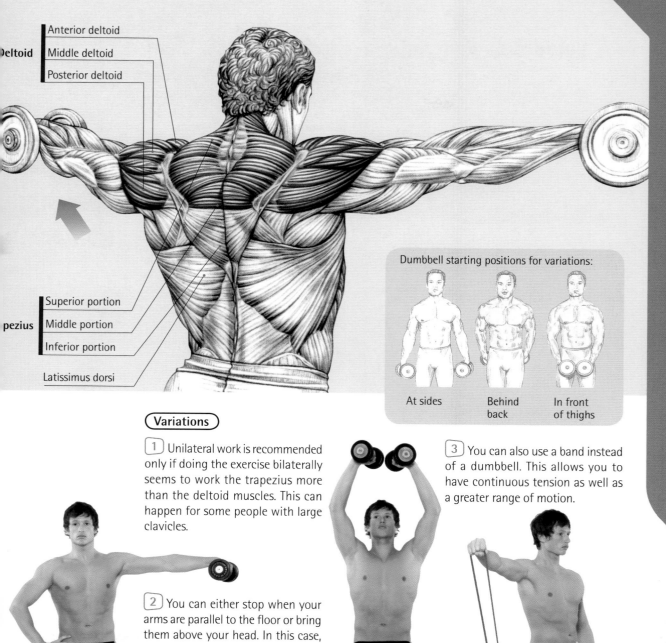

Anterior deltoid
Deltoid — Middle deltoid
Posterior deltoid

Superior portion
pezius — Middle portion
Inferior portion

Latissimus dorsi

Dumbbell starting positions for variations:

At sides | Behind back | In front of thighs

Variations

1 Unilateral work is recommended only if doing the exercise bilaterally seems to work the trapezius more than the deltoid muscles. This can happen for some people with large clavicles.

2 You can either stop when your arms are parallel to the floor or bring them above your head. In this case, the lateral part of the shoulder works less; the trapezius and the front of the shoulder take over. This greater range of motion means you will not be able to lift as much weight, but it will result in a more intense burn. Let your muscle sensations guide you in determining how high to lift your arms.

3 You can also use a band instead of a dumbbell. This allows you to have continuous tension as well as a greater range of motion.

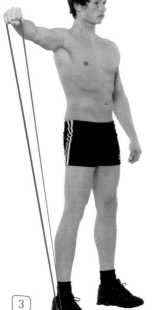

1

2

3

101

/// Lying One-Arm Lateral Raise

This is an isolation exercise for the lateral or back of the deltoid depending on the version you choose. The exercise must be done unilaterally.

For the lateral part of the shoulder:

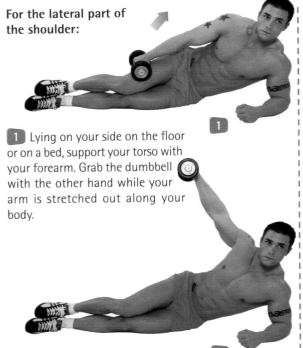

1 Lying on your side on the floor or on a bed, support your torso with your forearm. Grab the dumbbell with the other hand while your arm is stretched out along your body.

2 Lift the weight with your hand in the neutral position (thumb facing forward) and keep the arm very straight. Stop before the arm is perpendicular to the floor. The exercise is more difficult this way than when you are standing up.

For the back part of the shoulder:

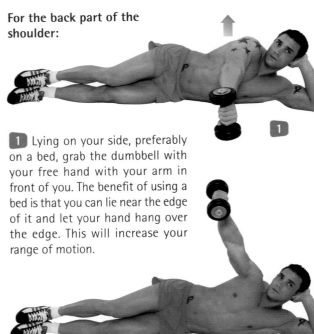

1 Lying on your side, preferably on a bed, grab the dumbbell with your free hand with your arm in front of you. The benefit of using a bed is that you can lie near the edge of it and let your hand hang over the edge. This will increase your range of motion.

2 Lift the weight with your hand in the neutral position (thumb toward the floor) and keep the arm very straight. Stop before the arm is perpendicular to the floor. In this way the exercise isolates the back of the shoulder better than with bent-over lateral raises (see page 104) since you can cheat by moving your torso. The stretching is much better and guarantees some aches and pains in the days that follow.

ADVANTAGES

If you have trouble feeling the work in your shoulder, especially in the back, then you should try this exercise. After several weeks of doing this exercise, you will learn to feel and better isolate these parts of the deltoid that are so difficult to work.

- - - - - - - - - - - - - - - - - -

Since this exercise has to be done unilaterally, it takes more time.

DISADVANTAGES

HELPFUL HINTS
The goal here is not to lift heavy weights. The lying position allows you to strictly isolate the movement. You must keep the arm straight for most of the exercise. At failure, you can bend it a little so that you can do a few more repetitions.

NOTES
Tapering sets is very appropriate for this exercise.

SHOULDERS

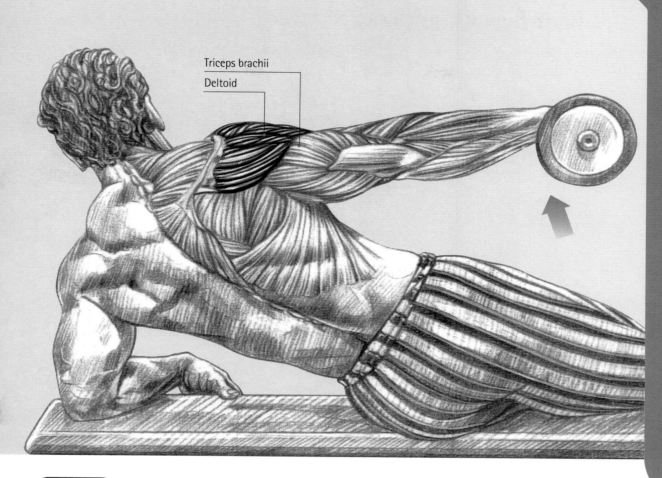

Triceps brachii

Deltoid

Variations

1 Ideally, you should do the follow-ing superset. Begin with the lying version.

2 At failure, stand up and finish the exercise while standing or bent over. You should be able to do a few more repetitions this way so that you truly exhaust the muscle.

! If you are lying on a bed, you need a firm mattress so that you can keep your back straight.

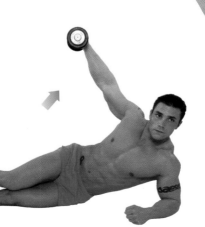

1

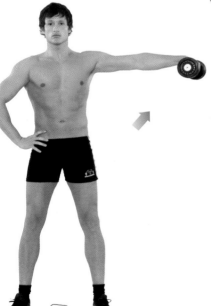

2

/// Bent-Over Lateral Raise

This is an isolation exercise for the back of the shoulders, but it also works the trapezius muscles and a part of the back. Though it can be done unilaterally, this may not be the best way to do the exercise.

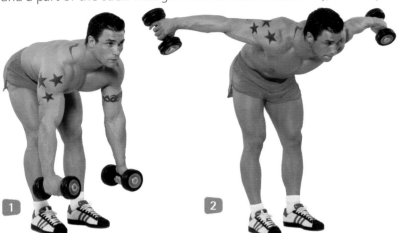

❗ The fact that you are bending over during this exercise puts your back in a very vulnerable position. To ease the burden on your lower back, press your rib cage against your thighs. During the entire exercise, keep the low back very straight.

1 Leaning forward, your torso should be near a 90-degree angle to the floor. Grab the dumbbells using a pronated grip (thumbs toward one another).

2 Lift your arms to the sides as high as possible while keeping them very straight. Hold the contracted position for one to two seconds before lowering the weights.

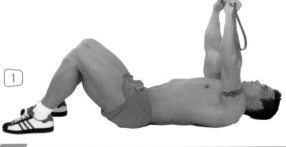

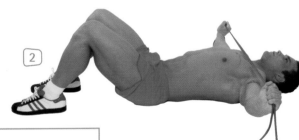

HELPFUL HINTS

Raise your arms straight up to your sides. It is easier to let your arms drift backward. In this position, you will be able to use heavier weights, but you will not isolate the back of the shoulders nearly as well. Keep your head very straight and look straight ahead with your gaze slightly upward so that you keep your back very straight.

If you want to work unilaterally, it is better to do the exercise on page 102.

NOTES

As we saw in the introduction to this chapter, individuals often neglect the back of the shoulders. Though it is not required that you work the front of the shoulders every time you work your deltoids, it is imperative that you work the back of the shoulders. If you are working the back on a different day than you work your shoulders, you can do a few sets of bent-over lateral raises just after your back work as a kind of muscular recall.

(Variations)

1 Lie on your back. Grab a band with your arms stretched out in front of you (using a pronated grip: thumbs toward each other).

2 Using the back of your shoulders, lower your arms to the floor. This version has the added benefit of not putting pressure on your spinal column.

SHOULDERS

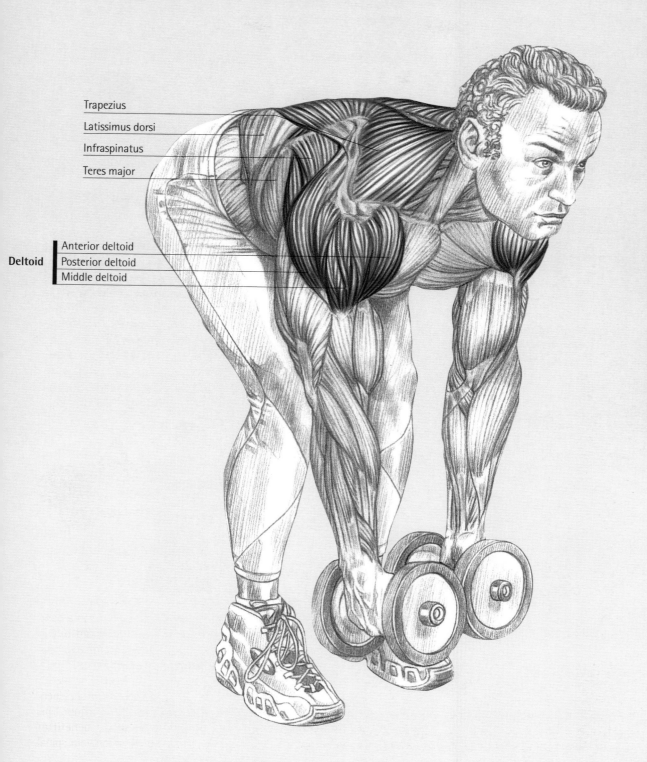

Trapezius

Latissimus dorsi

Infraspinatus

Teres major

Deltoid
Anterior deltoid
Posterior deltoid
Middle deltoid

/// Stretching the Shoulders

For the front of the shoulders:

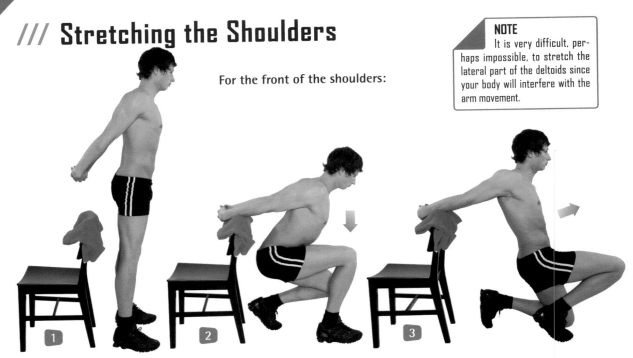

1 Stand with your hands clasped behind your back. Then put your hands on the back of a chair behind you. You can brace the chair with one of your feet so that it does not move.

2 Lean forward while lowering yourself. This will raise your arms behind you.

3 If you move forward, the stretch will be more intense. You can put a towel between your hands and the chair to prevent discomfort to your wrists.

For the back of the shoulders:

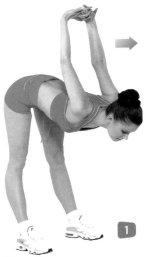

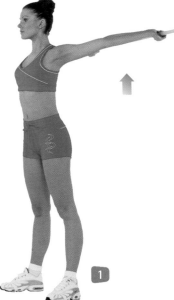

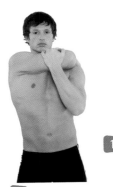

1 With your legs straight and your feet parallel, clasp your hands behind your thighs. Lean forward as you bring your arms up behind your shoulders. Bend your knees slightly and come back up by rolling through the spine.

1 Stand with your legs apart and your hands on either end of a weight bar.

Keep your arms straight and make a circle by bringing the bar above your head.

1 Stand with your right arm bent to 90 degrees and lift it to your neck. Rest the right hand on the left shoulder. Grab the right elbow with the left hand. Push your right arm toward your neck as much as you can. Hold the position and then repeat with the other arm.

When you become more flexible, you can press the elbow against a wall and let your body weight do the stretch.

SHOULDERS

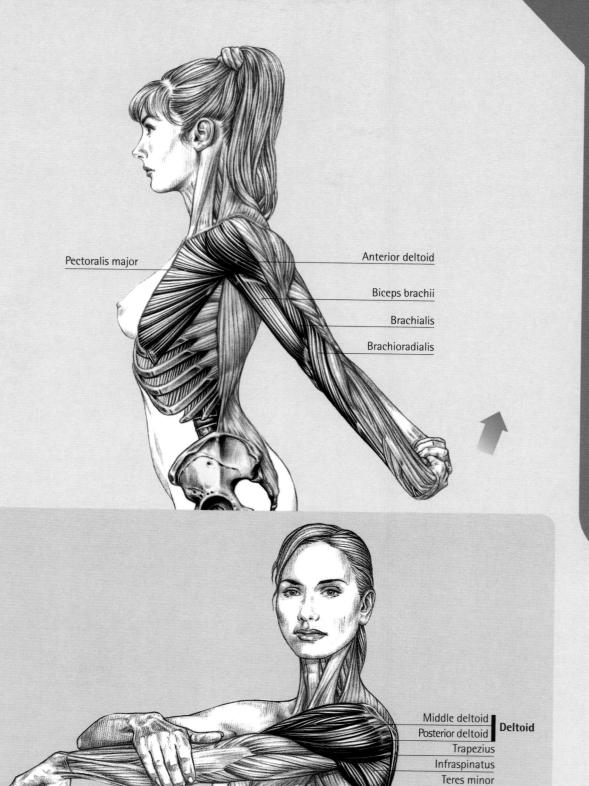

Pectoralis major

Anterior deltoid

Biceps brachii

Brachialis

Brachioradialis

Middle deltoid
Posterior deltoid **Deltoid**
Trapezius
Infraspinatus
Teres minor
Teres major

Infraspinatus

❚ Role of the Infraspinatus

The infraspinatus is one of the four muscles that make up the rotator cuff. There are four muscles (infraspinatus, supraspinatus, teres minor, and subscapularis) that surround the shoulder joint and hold it in place. As soon as you move the shoulder, the joint is inclined to dislocate.

It is clear that the rotator cuff muscles play a maintenance role. The rotator cuff is put to an abrupt test during almost all weight training exercises for the torso. It is no different in sports that involve the arms, such as swimming or shot put, for example.

It is easy to understand how this extreme work easily leads to injuries in the shoulder stabilizer muscles. These injuries are even more frequent since these four protective muscles are rather small. Of the four muscles, the infraspinatus is both the most used and the most fragile. This is why you must reinforce it by working it in a specific manner.

This work can be done in two ways:

1. During warm-up. All torso workouts begin with two to three light infraspinatus sets. This warm-up will prevent the muscle from being too cold during heavy sets. In addition, this regular work will also provide basic reinforcement that will prevent injuries.

2. At the end of a workout. In cases where the warm-up work was not enough or if you feel that your shoulder is unstable, more intense training is necessary. Most people do not realize that infraspinatus work is necessary until their shoulder is already causing them pain. But it is better to realize it too late than never to realize it at all. In this case, do three to five infraspinatus sets at the end of your torso workout. This specialization does not replace the infraspinatus warm-up sets.

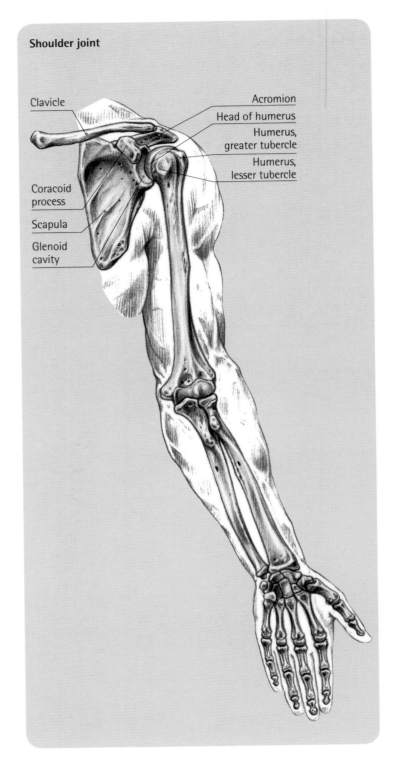

Shoulder joint

Clavicle

Coracoid process

Scapula

Glenoid cavity

Acromion

Head of humerus

Humerus, greater tubercle

Humerus, lesser tubercle

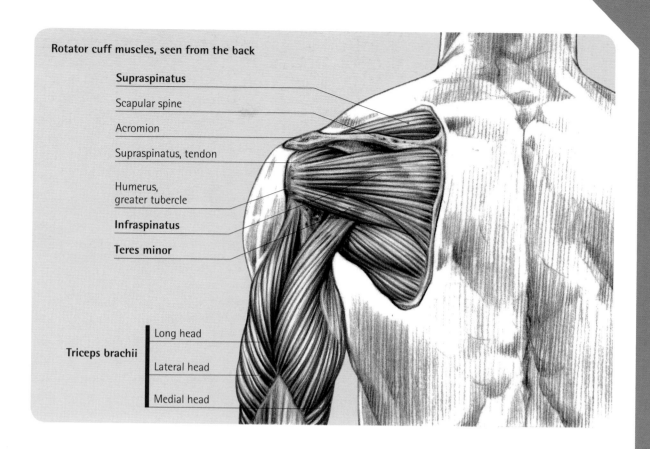

Rotator cuff muscles, seen from the back

Supraspinatus

Scapular spine

Acromion

Supraspinatus, tendon

Humerus,
greater tubercle

Infraspinatus

Teres minor

Triceps brachii
- Long head
- Lateral head
- Medial head

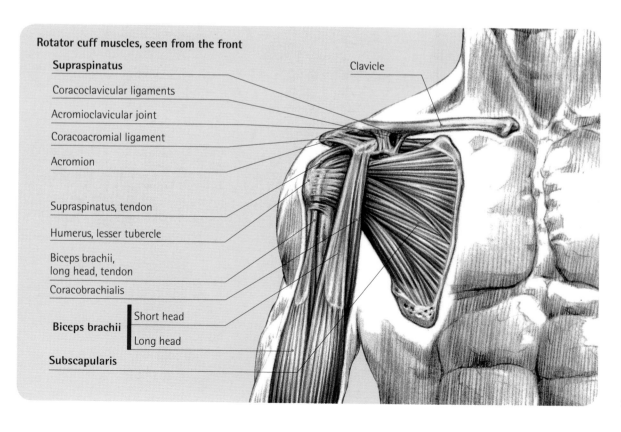

Rotator cuff muscles, seen from the front

Supraspinatus

Clavicle

Coracoclavicular ligaments

Acromioclavicular joint

Coracoacromial ligament

Acromion

Supraspinatus, tendon

Humerus, lesser tubercle

Biceps brachii,
long head, tendon

Coracobrachialis

Biceps brachii
- Short head
- Long head

Subscapularis

Shoulder Rotation With a Dumbbell

This is an isolation exercise for the infraspinatus. It must be done unilaterally.

TIP
Do at least 20 repetitions. You will be able to feel the work done by the infraspinatus better if you achieve burn during a long set.

! If you lower your arm too abruptly in the stretched position, you could tear your infraspinatus. You must do this exercise slowly and with great control in order to avoid injury.

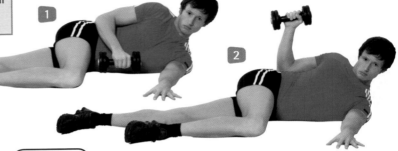

1 Lie on your left side on a bed or on the floor. Bend your right arm to 90 degrees while keeping the internal part of the biceps touching your torso.

2 With a dumbbell in hand and using a neutral grip (thumb toward your head), rotate your forearm as if you were hitchhiking. Stop just before your forearm is perpendicular to the floor. Then slowly lower your arm.

Variations

v You can change your hand position to see if you feel the exercise better with a supinated grip (pinkie finger toward the torso) or a pronated grip (thumb toward the torso).

HELPFUL HINTS
There is absolutely no reason to use a heavy weight in this exercise. Focus on doing the exercise well and feeling the infraspinatus work; neither of these is easy to do.

NOTES
A high volume of work (a large number of sets and workouts) must compensate for the low intensity of this exercise.

ADVANTAGES

Even if this exercise is not ideal, it is still better than nothing. You have to try to find the sensation of contraction during continuous tension rather than during performance.

The resistance the dumbbell provides is poorly adapted to the work required for the infraspinatus. Range of motion is reduced and tension is rather erratic. This can be traumatic for an already fragile muscle.

DISADVANTAGES

/// Stretching the Infraspinatus

To stretch your infraspinatus muscle, use the seated back stretch described on page 137.

SHOULDERS

/// Shoulder Rotation With a Band

1 Attach a band securely to an object at waist level on your right side. Stand with your feet slightly apart and bend your left arm 90 degrees while keeping the internal part of the biceps touching the torso. Grab the band using a neutral grip (thumb facing up).

2 Rotate your forearm as if you were hitchhiking. Inflate your rib cage so that you go as far as possible to the left. This inflation also allows for a better contraction of your infraspinatus muscle. Hold the contracted position for one to two seconds before breathing and bringing the forearm to the right. Stop the stretch the moment you feel your elbow lifting. Do at least 12 repetitions.

! Using a band is much less traumatic than using a dumbbell, so the risk of injury is less as well. However, you should still avoid any abrupt or exaggerated stretching.

▼ Pronated grip

▼ Supinated grip

ADVANTAGES

This exercise is the most efficient for warming up and strengthening the infraspinatus muscle.

- - - - - - - - - - - - - - - - - -

It is difficult to quantify the resistance provided by a band. If you don't have a way to measure this, it can make progress difficult.

DISADVANTAGES

(Variations)

v Try to change the hand position to see if you can feel the exercise better with a supinated grip (thumb toward the outside) or a pronated grip (thumb toward the torso).

You often see this exercise done with a dumbbell. Unfortunately, it is completely useless, because the resistance needs to come from the side and not from above, as is the case with weights.

SCULPT YOUR CHEST

▌Role of the Pectoralis Muscles

The pectoralis muscles allow you to move your arm forward when your arm must overcome resistance (for example, when pushing an opponent away).

The pectoralis muscles are therefore often used in combat sports, contact sports, and any sport that involves throwing. A kind of armor, they are to some degree the muscles of confrontation.

Aesthetically, they are highly sought after because their development is a sign of virility and power in men.

The pectoralis muscles are not commonly used in daily activities, so they are often underdeveloped. Beginning weight trainers may have trouble feeling these muscles working.

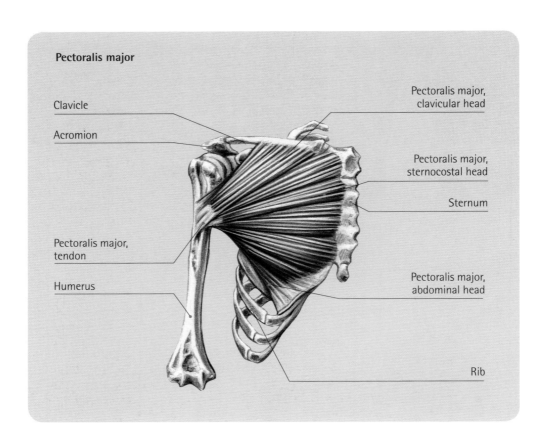

Pectoralis major

Clavicle

Acromion

Pectoralis major, tendon

Humerus

Pectoralis major, clavicular head

Pectoralis major, sternocostal head

Sternum

Pectoralis major, abdominal head

Rib

CHEST

/// Push-Up

This is a multijoint exercise for the chest, shoulders, and triceps.
Unilateral work is possible, but only for extremely light people.

1 Stretch out facing the floor with your hands on the floor. Your hands should be at least shoulder-width apart.

2 Straighten your arms to raise your body using your chest as much as you can. Once the arms are straight, lower yourself slowly back down.

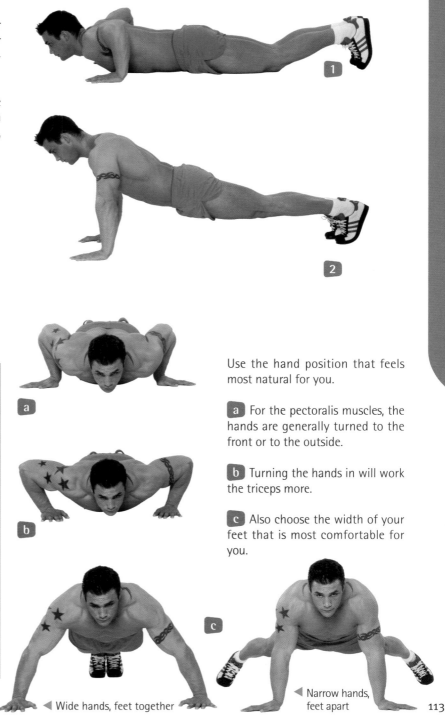

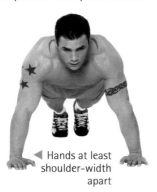

◄ Hands at least shoulder-width apart

HELPFUL HINTS

1. Wide hands. The farther apart your hands are, the more you will stretch the chest muscles. Not all of your tendons will appreciate this movement, though, especially if you have long forearms. However, once your arms are straight, the contraction shortens the chest muscles to a lesser degree.

2. Narrow hands. On the contrary, the closer together your hands are, the less stretch there will be. This is less risky for the pectoralis major tendon. There is greater shortening of the pectoralis muscles once the arm is straight. The only risk is that the triceps, which work more with narrow hands, will take over some of the work from the pectoralis muscles.

Use the hand position that feels most natural for you.

a For the pectoralis muscles, the hands are generally turned to the front or to the outside.

b Turning the hands in will work the triceps more.

c Also choose the width of your feet that is most comfortable for you.

◄ Wide hands, feet together

◄ Narrow hands, feet apart

113

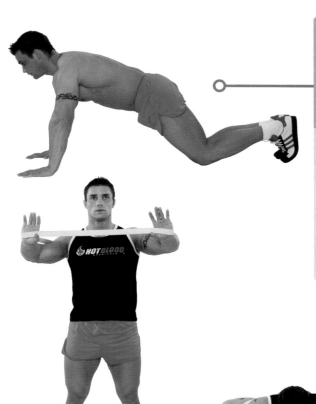

It is easy to vary resistance. If your body weight is too great, begin doing push-ups on your knees rather than on your feet so that you can gain strength. In the same way, at the end of a set in which you are doing push-ups from the feet, if you are not strong enough to do classic push-ups, continue doing the exercise on your knees so you can do a few more repetitions.

It is not easy to focus solely on the pectoralis muscles during push-ups. In addition, push-ups do not work well for every person's anatomy. If you have long arms, you will have difficulties without any guarantee of results. Push-ups are not the end goal. Weight training should not be a select club for people who can do push-ups or a circus for people to show off crazy push-up variations. The only goal is effective muscle work.

DISADVANTAGES

[1]

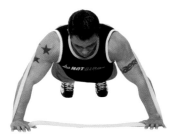

[1]

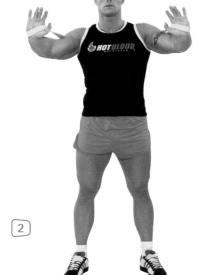

(**Variations**)

[1] To add resistance, use a band. Wrap it around your back and hold it in your hands. Begin with only one loop around your back.

The angle between the chest and the arms can vary. You can choose the more comfortable position: either having your hands under your shoulders or having them under your chest.

[2]

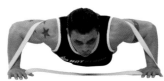

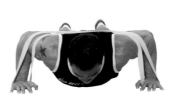

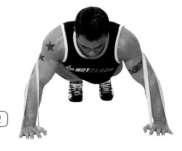

[2]

[2] When you are stronger, you can loop the band twice around your back.

CHEST

114

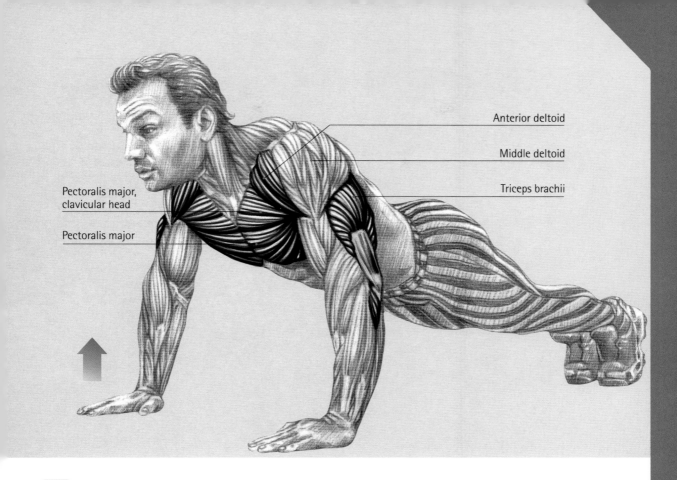

Anterior deltoid

Middle deltoid

Triceps brachii

Pectoralis major, clavicular head

Pectoralis major

NOTES

Push-ups draw a circular arc with the body: Your body does not come up parallel to the floor. The head moves much more than the legs. If you cannot feel this rotation, you can put heavy phone books under your thighs or knees. The exercise will be easier (the closer the phone books are to your torso, the easier the exercise will be) but also more natural for the joints and muscles. If you do not feel your muscles working during classic push-ups, this elevated version will certainly help you.

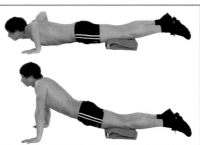

! All wrists are not made to be bent at a 90-degree angle. So that you do not damage your wrists for no reason, you can put phone books on the floor. Special push-up bars are also available in sporting goods stores. They increase the range of motion of the exercise while preventing too much twisting (excessive twisting is not natural for the wrists).

Arching your back will make this exercise easier, but it could compromise your spine unnecessarily.

TIP

One way to quickly gain strength in multijoint exercises for the pectoralis muscles is to do a biceps set (without forcing things too much) between two sets of push-ups or bench presses. Moderate biceps work accelerates the recovery of the triceps, preventing premature fatigue.

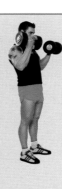

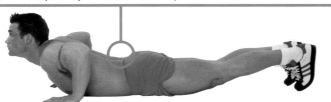

115

/// Bench Press With Dumbbells

This is a multijoint exercise for the chest, shoulders, and triceps. Unilateral work is possible, but it may not be useful for a beginner because the exercise becomes rather unstable.

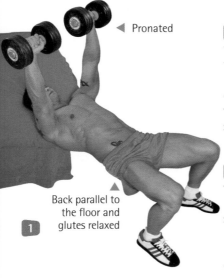

◄ Pronated

▲ Back parallel to the floor and glutes relaxed

[1]

Dumbbells at upper chest ▼

▲ Elbows spread out

[2]

! Pay attention when you lift the dumbbells from the floor to your starting position. Place the weights on your thighs, arms bent, so that you can move with your back well protected. In the same way, when you lay the weights back down, do not stretch out your arms to drop the weights because you could tear your biceps.

[1] Lying with your back on the floor or on the corner of a bed, bring the dumbbells to your shoulders in a pronated grip (thumbs toward each other). Straighten your arms using your chest muscles. Dumbbells should touch each other at the height of the movement.

[2] Lower the weight by bending your arms and moving the dumbbells apart. The ending point can be somewhere between the upper chest (shoulder level) and the lower chest (nipple level). At first, you should determine the ending point based on what feels most natural for you. Later, you can choose the ending point based on your goals. Starting at the upper chest will work the upper part of the pectoralis major muscle more; starting at the lower chest will work the lower part of the muscle more.

Variations

[1] The orientation of the hands and elbows can vary. Keeping the elbows along the body and the hands in a neutral position (thumbs toward the head) stretches the pectoralis major less and forces the shoulders to work more.

Spreading the elbows as far away from the body as possible and using a pronated grip (thumbs facing each other) greatly stretches the chest muscles at the bottom of the movement. The risk of tearing the pectoralis major is greater, but the muscle is worked much harder. You must determine which position works your muscles the most.

Incline bench press

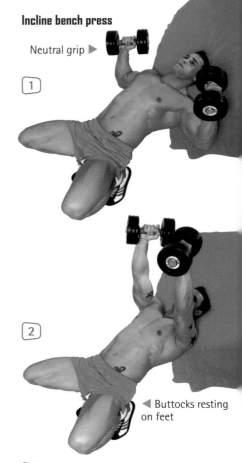

Neutral grip ►

[1]

[2]

◄ Buttocks resting on feet

[2] On the corner of the bed, instead of keeping your torso parallel to the floor, you can lower your buttocks to rest on your heels. This inclined position will force the upper-chest muscles to work more.

[3] You can also do the bench press for the chest while standing up with a band wrapped around your back and held in both hands. Push on the band with one or both arms. This version is very useful for combat sports such as boxing.

CHEST

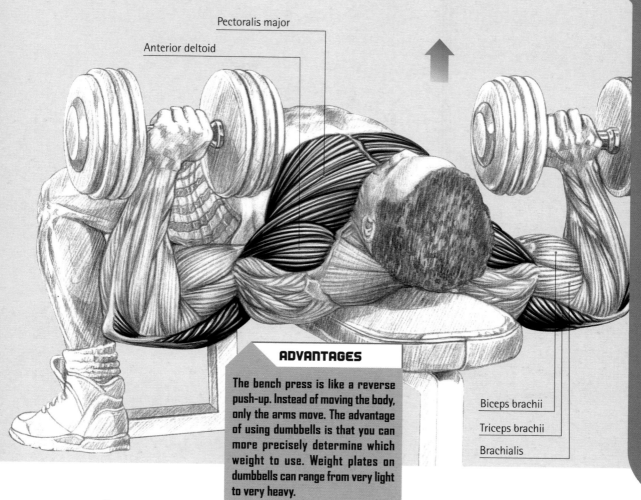

Anterior deltoid

Pectoralis major

Biceps brachii

Triceps brachii

Brachialis

ADVANTAGES

The bench press is like a reverse push-up. Instead of moving the body, only the arms move. The advantage of using dumbbells is that you can more precisely determine which weight to use. Weight plates on dumbbells can range from very light to very heavy.

The freedom of movement of the arms requires you to gain better muscle control. This mastery can be difficult to acquire for some beginners. Push-ups are not as difficult to perform. At first, push-ups will be easier to do than bench presses. Moreover, this freedom of arm movement is more representative of what is required in various sports. Because of the difficulty in mastering this movement, the bench press is a better exercise for athletes than push-ups.

DISADVANTAGES

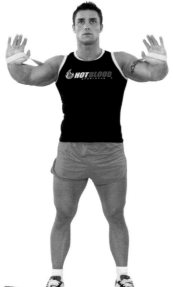

HELPFUL HINTS
The range of motion for this exercise is limited when it is performed on the floor. Lying on the corner of a bed is more comfortable and lets you have a complete range of motion. It will take some time for you to learn to master this exercise completely. You should begin with a light weight so that you can get used to the exercise.

NOTES
When you are on the edge of the bed, stabilize yourself using your legs. Pushing on your thighs will give you strength. Be certain that your bed will not move or tip over when you lie down on its corner.

3

/// Dumbbell Chest Fly

This is an isolation exercise for the chest and the shoulders. Though you could work unilaterally, you should not do so.

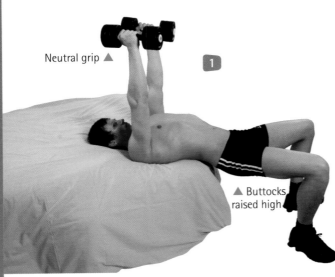

Neutral grip ▲

1

▲ Buttocks raised high

HELPFUL HINTS

The dumbbells do not have to touch at the top of the movement. In fact, there is little resistance at the height of the exercise. If you cannot feel your chest muscles when your arms are up, it is better to work under continuous tension. Stop when you are 75 percent of the way through the movement rather than perform the complete movement.

NOTES

One possible combination is to begin with chest flys. At failure, bend your arms more and more to transform the exercise into a bench press with dumbbells so that you can do more repetitions.

! Never straighten your arms in order to put the weights back on the floor because you could tear your biceps. In the same way, you should never straighten your arms completely during the exercise.

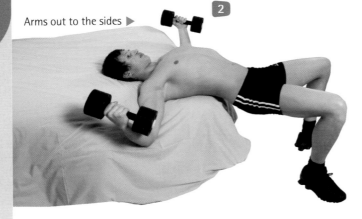

Arms out to the sides ▶

2

ADVANTAGES

Chest flys provide a good stretch for the pectoralis muscles. And, unlike bench presses, the triceps muscles are not involved, which means they will not get tired before the pectoralis muscles do.

It can be difficult to focus the work only on the pectoralis muscles and not the shoulders. Also, since almost no resistance exists at the top of the movement, it can be difficult to feel the pectoralis muscles contract.

DISADVANTAGES

1 Lie on the floor or on the corner of a bed. Grab two dumbbells and bring them to your shoulders in a neutral hand grip (thumbs pointing up). Straighten your arms in front of you as if you were doing a bench press.

2 Once in position, lower your arms to your sides while keeping them semistraight. Once your arms are at the same level, bring the dumbbells together using your chest muscles. Lower the weights by moving the dumbbells apart without bending your arms too much.

CHEST

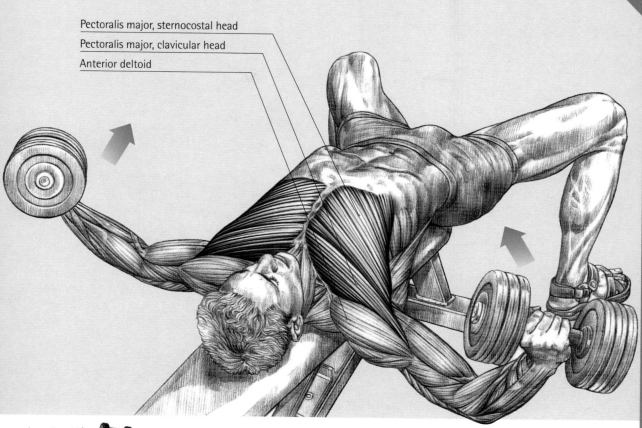

Pectoralis major, sternocostal head
Pectoralis major, clavicular head
Anterior deltoid

Arms in a V ▶

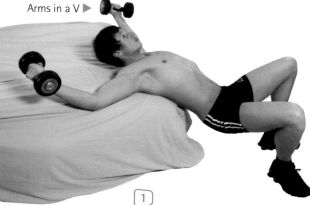

1

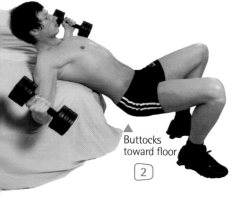

Buttocks
toward floor

2

Variations

You can rotate your wrists so that you can feel the pectoralis muscles contracting more. In the first version, the closer your hands are together, the more you will turn your pinkie fingers toward each other. The contraction will be more pronounced in the lower-pectoralis muscles.

In the second version, the closer your hands are together, the more you will turn your thumbs toward each other. The contraction will be more pronounced in the upper-pectoralis muscles and shoulders.

1 Instead of lowering your arms to your sides, you can lower them in a V shape or much closer to your head. This creates a hybrid exercise between chest flys and pull-overs. Some people will be able to feel the exercise more this way. However, you have to use much lighter weights because the movement is more difficult and the risk of tearing a muscle is much greater.

2 If you are on the corner of the bed, you can lower your buttocks toward the floor instead of keeping your torso parallel to it. This inclined position forces the upper-pectoralis muscles to work much harder.

119

/// Straight-Arm Pullover

This is an isolation exercise for the chest and, to a lesser extent, the latissimus dorsi and the triceps. Unilateral work is possible but not desirable.

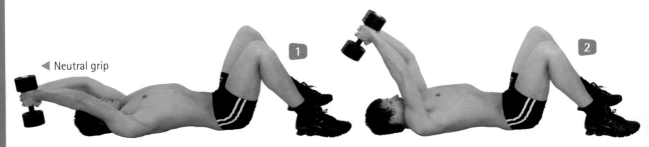

◀ Neutral grip

1 Lie on your back either on the floor or on a bed (preferred). In the latter case, your head should be just on the edge of the bed so that your arms can hang freely. This will give you a greater range of motion and a better stretch. Holding a dumbbell with both hands in a neutral grip (thumbs toward the floor), straighten your arms above your head.

2 Keep your arms straight and lower them behind your head. When your arms are extended from your body, raise them back up using the strength of your pectoralis muscles. Stop the movement when the dumbbell is above your head and then lower it again.

(**Variations**)

v Instead of using a single dumbbell, you can hold one dumbbell in each hand. In this case, the exercise is much harder because better muscle control is required in order to move two dumbbells at the same time. One possible combination is to begin with pullovers using two weights. At failure, change the exercise to chest flys so that you can get more repetitions as well as a different stretch of the pectoralis muscles.

During tapering, you can begin the pullover with two dumbbells. At failure, set one weight down and continue the exercise with a single dumbbell.

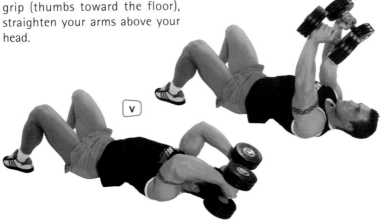

! The straight-arm pullover puts the shoulder joints in a relatively precarious position, so you must not use too heavy a weight. Increase the number of repetitions rather than increase the weight. Also, be sure that the weights are securely attached to the bar because you do not want them to fall off when the bar is going past your face.

ADVANTAGES

This exercise stretches the pectoralis muscles and shoulders simultaneously (two groups that tend to lose flexibility during weight training).

Some people cannot feel their pectoralis muscles working during this exercise. Their back muscles are doing most of the work.

DISADVANTAGES

HELPFUL HINTS
You can very slightly bend your arms to increase the stretch, but if you bend them too much, the work will be done more and more by the back muscles and less and less by the pectoralis muscles.

NOTES
You can use the pullover to open up the rib cage. However, there are more effective stretching exercises that will accomplish the same thing.

CHEST

120

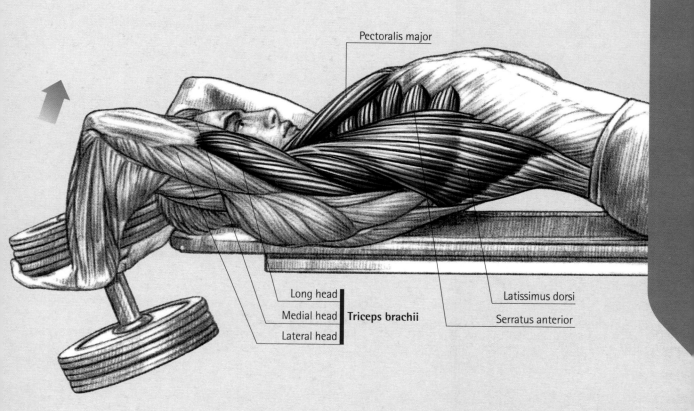

Pectoralis major

Long head
Medial head **Triceps brachii**
Lateral head

Latissimus dorsi
Serratus anterior

/// Crossover With a Band

This is an isolation exercise for the chest and the shoulders.
It is best to do this exercise unilaterally.

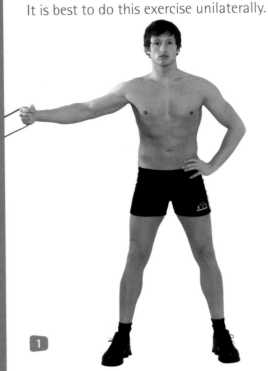

1

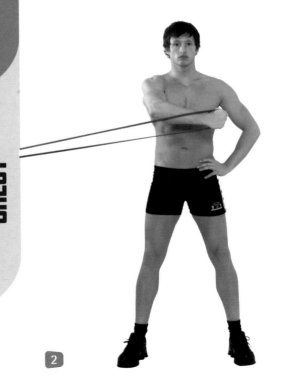

2

1 Attach your band to a fixed point at about waist level (for example, you could attach it to your pull-up bar or to a doorknob). Lengthen or shorten the band to reach the desired tension. While standing, hold the other end of the band in your right hand in a neutral grip (thumb facing forward or toward the ceiling, depending on your arm position).

2 Keeping your arm almost straight, bring it toward your torso using the strength of your chest muscles. Maintain the contracted position for one second before returning to the starting position. When you have finished with the right arm, move immediately to the left arm, and so on.

HELPFUL HINTS
To really work your chest muscles, you must do this exercise slowly and with continuous tension. It becomes much easier if you bend your arm; this is why you need to keep your arm almost straight. When you reach failure, you can always bend the arm a little bit so that you can do a few more repetitions.

! Never completely straighten your arm during this exercise, because you could tear your biceps muscle. Do not bend your arm too much, either, because then you will not feel the exercise very much.

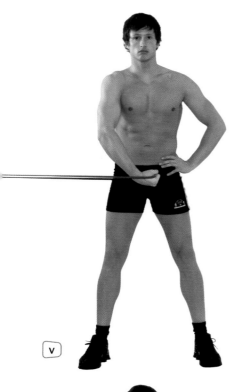

Variations

v You can also bring the arm toward your abdomen or your head (or anywhere else between these two points) in order to change the angle at which the pectoralis muscles work. In fact, the pectoralis are muscles that should be worked at different angles.

Instead of attaching the band to a fixed point, step on it with your right foot when you are working your right side. Lift your hand with your arm straight up to your eye level.

NOTES

If you have trouble feeling your pectoralis muscles during multijoint exercises, you can learn to feel their contractions using this exercise. After two or three weeks of working with a band, you will have better sensations during other pectoralis muscle exercises.

v

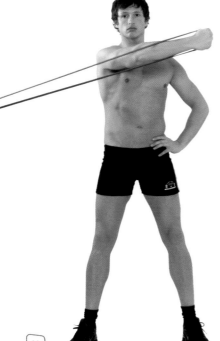

v

ADVANTAGES

This exercise resembles a chest fly, but the advantage of using a band is that it provides resistance during the entire exercise and not just during half of it, as when you use dumbbells.

You will lose a certain amount of time during the workout since this exercise must be done unilaterally.

DISADVANTAGES

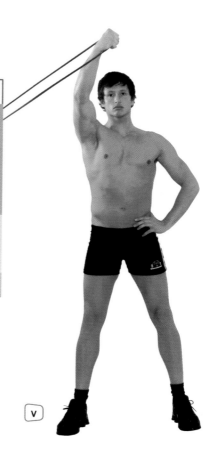

v

123

/// Plyometric Exercises for the Pectorals

Hands shoulder-width apart
▼

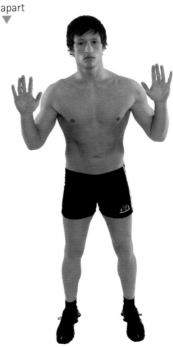

▲
Bent arms

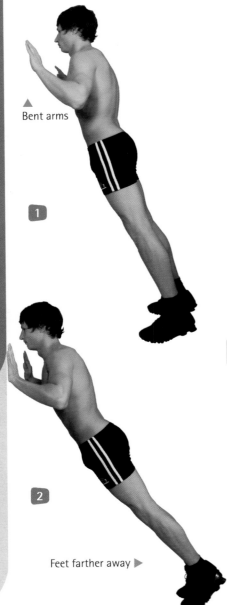

1

2

Feet farther away ▶

The main plyometric exercise for the pectoralis muscles is push-ups against a wall or on the floor. Your hands should be about shoulder-width apart. Begin with the version where you push against a wall so that you can get used to the exercise.

1 Standing up facing a wall, let your body fall toward the wall.

2 At the last moment, use your arms to push off so that you do not hit the wall. The farther you are away from the wall, the more difficult the exercise becomes.

HELPFUL HINTS
If you bend your arms, the exercise will be harder. The easiest thing to do would be to keep your arms straight, but then the exercise would be dangerous. So you must always keep your arms slightly bent.

NOTES
As with all plyometric exercises, contact time should be minimal. Once the hands touch the wall or the floor, you must push off immediately.

(**Variations**)

Once you are comfortable with the upright version close to the wall, you should move farther and farther away. When you feel ready, try the lying version on your knees. After that, you can try the regular version.

ADVANTAGES

This exercise will give you power in all sports in which you need to push an opponent or an object, including rugby, martial arts, volleyball, basketball, and shot put.

Do not overestimate your strength or you could hit your head.

DISADVANTAGES

! This exercise can be hard on your elbows and shoulders.

CHEST

/// Stretching the Pectorals

1 Stand in a doorway (or beside another fixed point) and place your right arm, bent to 90 degrees, against the door frame. Support yourself against the frame using your hand and elbow. Take a small step forward and lean forward.

Once you are finished stretching the pectoralis major, move on to your left arm. Though it is possible to stretch both arms at the same time, if you do this, then the range of motion will be much smaller. Stretch both arms at the same time during your first month of training. After this, begin doing the unilateral version.

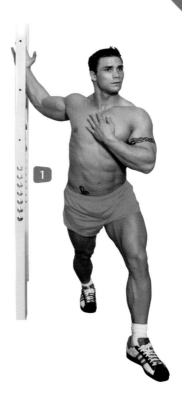

/// Stretching the Rib Cage

1 Stand up behind a fixed point at about chest height (near furniture or a door frame). Put both hands around this point with your thumbs turned toward each other, practically touching. Using this object, push on your arms and take a deep breath so that you inflate your rib cage to its maximum. You should see your rib cage opening up. Try to squeeze your shoulder blades together.

2 Exhale all the air so that you deflate the rib cage. Repeat this breathing pattern several times. You will quickly see that it becomes ever easier to expand your rib cage because you gain flexibility and mobility in your sides.

Unlike a pullover exercise where it is difficult to expand the rib cage fully, there is no dangerous tension applied to the shoulders during this stretch.

This exercise improves the placement of the torso during exercises for the chest and back. It is also helpful in increasing endurance because of the respiratory muscles' work. See page 218 for more details about this.

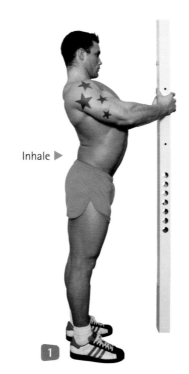

Inhale ▶

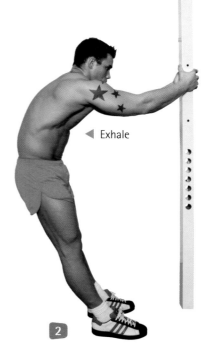

◀ Exhale

STRENGTHEN YOUR NECK

▌Role of the Neck Muscles

The muscles of the neck have three purposes:

1 These muscles, of course, ensure the mobility of the neck. They allow you to turn your head from left to right and from high to low. But because of its great mobility as well as the heavy weight of the head, the cervical spine takes a beating in many sports.

2 The second role of the neck muscles is therefore to protect the integrity of the cervical vertebrae in case of a shock. This is why it is important for athletes to work their neck muscles.

3 Aesthetically, a large neck is always impressive. A good example of this is champion boxers. This leads us to the third role of the neck: to intimidate adversaries with its size.

A complete program for the neck must include an exercise that works the muscles in these locations:
> ➤ The back of the neck (extensor muscles)
> ➤ The front of the neck (flexor muscles)
> ➤ The sides of the neck (rotator muscles)

We have assembled the best exercise for each of these three parts of the neck.

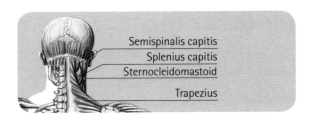

Semispinalis capitis
Splenius capitis
Sternocleidomastoid
Trapezius

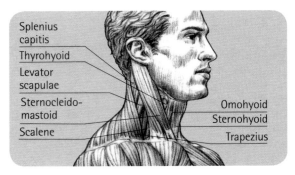

Splenius capitis
Thyrohyoid
Levator scapulae
Sternocleido-mastoid
Scalene
Omohyoid
Sternohyoid
Trapezius

! The cervical vertebrae are very small, but they have great mobility, so it is extremely easy to injure them. The purpose of weight training is to strengthen the neck muscles so that they will protect the cervical vertebrae during contact with opponents or the ground. But you must not lose sight of the fact that you can do just as much damage to your cervical spine with the weight training exercises themselves. So that you do not to work against your goals, you must perform neck exercises in a very controlled fashion and preferably in long sets so that you do not compress the cervical vertebrae (which you are trying to protect).

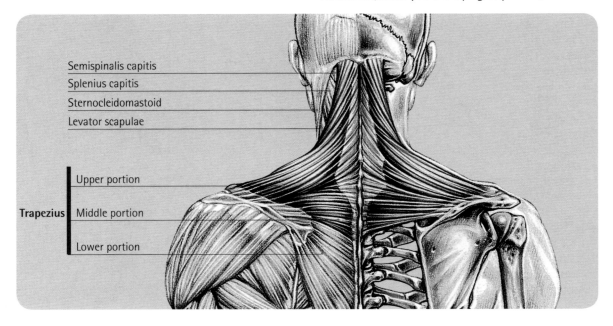

Semispinalis capitis
Splenius capitis
Sternocleidomastoid
Levator scapulae

Trapezius — Upper portion
Middle portion
Lower portion

/// Neck Extension

This is an isolation exercise for the muscles at the back of the neck. It cannot be done unilaterally.

1 While sitting or standing, intertwine your fingers and put your hands behind your head. Your hands provide the resistance in this exercise.

2 Using the strength in your neck, push your hands as far back as possible. Hold the contracted position for three to four seconds. Slowly push your head back to the front with your hands while resisting with your neck.

Variations

To avoid movement if your neck is already sore, you can do this exercise in an isometric (static) way. Lie flat on your back on a bed and then push your head down as far as possible into the mattress. Hold that position for 10 seconds and then relax for a few seconds. Repeat until fatigued.

! At no time should you apply pressure toward the floor with your hands, because this could compress the cervical vertebrae.

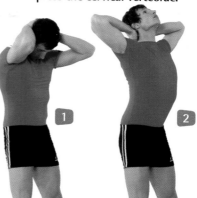

HELPFUL HINTS
Do not push your head too far down in the stretched position. The chin should not go much past the level where it is parallel to the floor.

NOTES
It is better to do neck exercises at the end of a workout because a tired neck could interfere with the proper training of other muscles. Athletes prefer to work on the neck while standing rather than while sitting because the muscles at the back of the neck work more while in a standing position.

ADVANTAGES

This body-weight movement works the neck without squishing the cervical spine, as can happen with weight training machines for the neck.

- -

Moving the neck in this way can cause vertigo. This is why you must do the exercise very slowly and under continuous tension. If you have vertigo, try the exercise with your eyes closed to see if this solves the problem.

DISADVANTAGES

/// Neck Flexion

This is an isolation exercise for the muscles in the front of the neck. It cannot be done unilaterally.

! To avoid pressure on the cervical spine, be careful not to lift the head too high in the air.

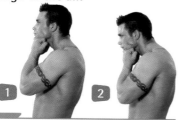

1 Standing or sitting, bring your fists together under your chin.

2 Using your neck, push on your fists as far forward as you can. Hold the contracted position for three to four seconds. Slowly bring your head back up using the fists while resisting the movement with your neck.

Variations

To avoid all movement, you can do this exercise isometrically. Place your fists between your chest and neck. Squeeze your neck muscles as hard as possible. Hold the position for 10 seconds and then relax for a few seconds. Repeat until fatigued.

ADVANTAGES

This body-weight movement works the neck while decompressing the cervical spine, which is a good thing to do at the end of a workout, particularly if you have just worked the trapezius muscles.

- -

It is difficult to evaluate the resistance that you are placing on your muscles. For this reason, gauging your progress is more difficult.

DISADVANTAGES

HELPFUL HINTS
Do not bring your head up too high in the stretched position. It is best if your chin does not go much beyond the level where it is parallel to the floor.

NOTES
You can combine neck flexion exercises with neck extensions in supersets without rest breaks.

/// Lateral Neck Extension

This is an isolation exercise for the muscles on the side of the neck.
This exercise must be done unilaterally.

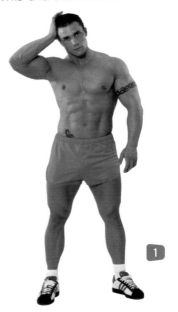

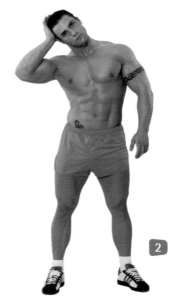

! Lateral work is the most dangerous type of exercise for the neck. Be satisfied with a very small range of motion. If you stretch your neck, do so with caution.

1 Stand or sit and put the palm of your right hand above your right ear.

2 Use the strength of your neck to push your hand as far as possible toward the right. Hold the contracted position for three to four seconds. Slowly bring the head back to the correct position by pushing with the hand while resisting with your neck. Once you have worked the right side, move immediately to the left side.

Variations

You can do this exercise while lying on your side and using only the weight of the head. You can also do it isometrically by maintaining the contracted position for 10 seconds each set without moving your head. Take a brief rest and repeat the move until fatigued.

ADVANTAGES

This exercise works the protective muscles of the neck, which is normally difficult to do.

- - - - - - - - - - - - - - - - - - -

Any sudden movement could injure the cervical spine. Remain focused throughout this exercise.

DISADVANTAGES

HELPFUL HINTS
Do not overwork the range of motion in your neck, especially in the stretched position.

NOTES
Work very slowly, maintaining continuous tension, almost in an isometric fashion.

NECK

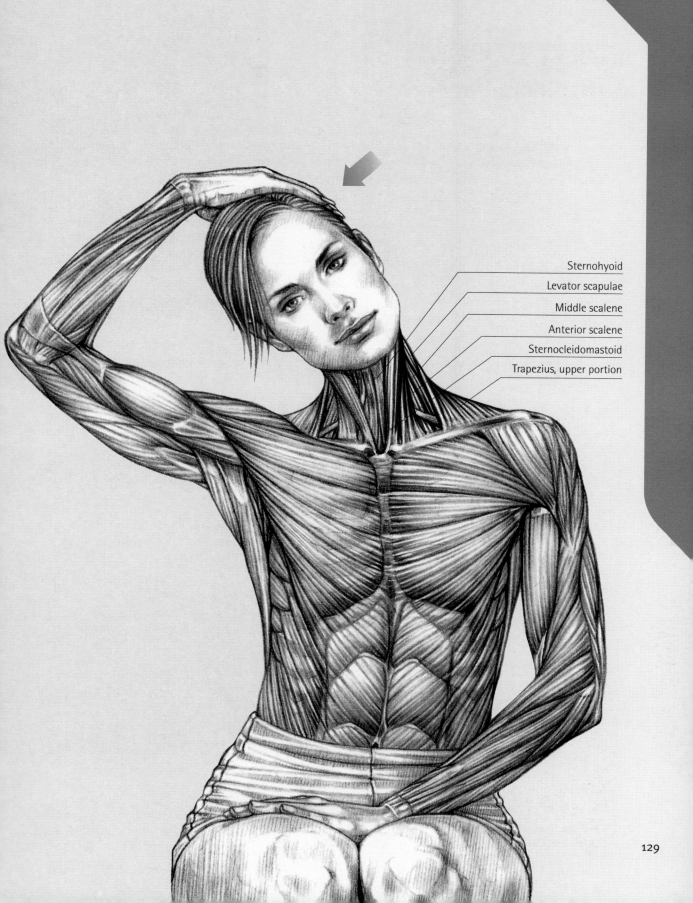

Sternohyoid

Levator scapulae

Middle scalene

Anterior scalene

Sternocleidomastoid

Trapezius, upper portion

SCULPT YOUR BACK
Latissimus Dorsi

▍Role of the Latissimus Dorsi

The latissimus dorsi muscles cover almost the entire back. They give the torso its V shape. Anatomically, they are responsible for pulling the arms behind the body. In this task, they are aided by the back of the shoulders, the biceps, and the long heads of the triceps. The work of the latissimus dorsi muscles is the opposite of the work done by the pectoralis muscles and the front of the shoulders, so these are antagonistic muscles.

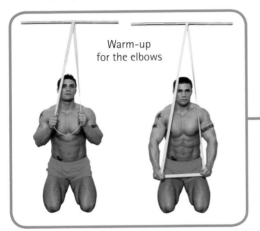

Warm-up
for the elbows

! Before working your back, be sure that you have really warmed up the elbows through some triceps work. As we have just seen, the triceps participate actively in all back work. An elbow that is cold when you begin a heavy back exercise will not necessarily be painful. But when you begin heavy triceps work, you may notice pain. This is why people do not always realize they have injured an elbow doing back exercises and not directly through triceps exercises.

BACK

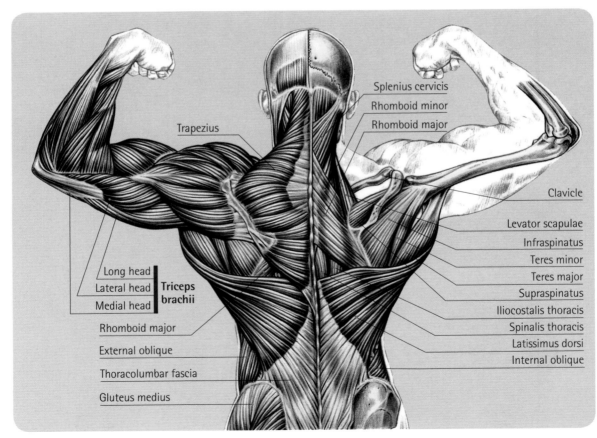

Trapezius

Splenius cervicis
Rhomboid minor
Rhomboid major

Clavicle

Levator scapulae
Infraspinatus
Teres minor
Teres major
Supraspinatus
Iliocostalis thoracis
Spinalis thoracis
Latissimus dorsi
Internal oblique

Long head
Lateral head — **Triceps brachii**
Medial head
Rhomboid major
External oblique
Thoracolumbar fascia
Gluteus medius

130

/// Chin-Up

This is a multijoint exercise for the back muscles as well as for the biceps, a part of the triceps, and the forearms. Unilateral work is nearly impossible except for very slight people.

▼ Supination

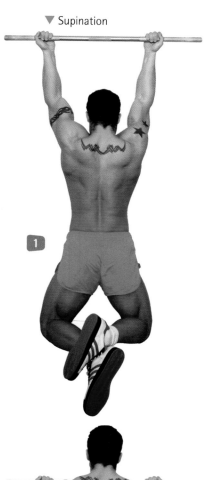

1 Grab the bar with supinated hands (pinkie fingers facing each other). Your hands should be about shoulder-width apart. Pull your feet up behind you so that the calves and thighs form a 90-degree angle. Cross your legs so that the right foot pushes against the left ankle.

2 Pull yourself using the strength of your back so that your forehead comes up to the level of the bar. If you are strong enough, bring your chin just to the bar while tilting your head back. If you are very strong, pull up to your neck, keeping your head tilted backward. Maintain the contracted position for one second before slowly coming down. Do not straighten the arms out completely. In this way you will maintain continuous tension and prevent injuries.

HELPFUL HINTS
Be sure that you have a good grip on the bar. To do this, put your thumb on your index finger (and your middle finger if your fingers are large enough) to support your fingers' hold on the bar.

At all times, keep your body straight by squeezing your buttocks together and pushing the right foot against the left ankle. This rigidity will help you avoid any swaying.

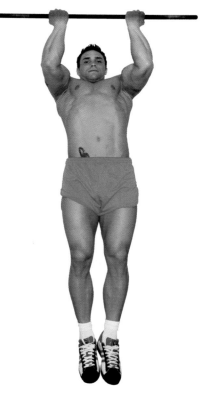

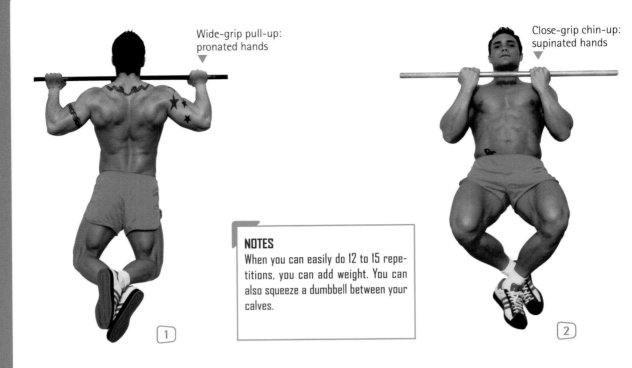

Wide-grip pull-up: pronated hands

Close-grip chin-up: supinated hands

1

2

NOTES
When you can easily do 12 to 15 repetitions, you can add weight. You can also squeeze a dumbbell between your calves.

Variations

1 Vary the position of your hands until you find what works best for you. You can also use a pronated grip (thumbs facing each other) to change the angle of attack for this exercise.

You have the option of bringing the bar in front of or behind the head. This latter version is the most difficult and most traumatizing to the shoulder joints.

2 You can use a close grip with supinated hands (pinkie fingers toward each other) as you would for working the biceps. The exercise is easier this way, but the biceps work more than they would with a wider grip. A supinated close grip can be used advantageously by beginners who cannot pull themselves up any other way.

If you cannot do one repetition, even with a supinated close grip, you will find a negative method on page 48 that will help you quickly gain strength.

page 48

ADVANTAGES

In very little time, chin-ups work a very large section of the muscles in the torso. There is nothing better than chin-ups to make your back bigger.

- - - - - - - - - - - - - - - - -

Everyone is unfortunately not able to pull themselves up using the horizontal bar, which can be frustrating.

DISADVANTAGES

! As with all pull-up exercises, you should never straighten your arms completely. This places the biceps and shoulders in a vulnerable position where something could tear. If you ever straighten your arms in order to rest between two repetitions, do not begin again abruptly with a jerky movement. Your shoulder ligaments are in a precarious position when you are hanging with straight arms, and you do not want to pull anything. The idea with pull-up exercises is to maintain continuous tension during the entire stretching part of the exercise.

BACK

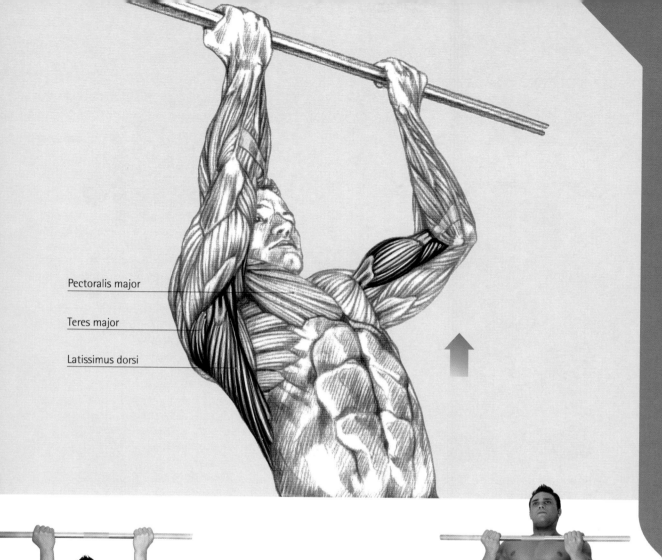

Pectoralis major

Teres major

Latissimus dorsi

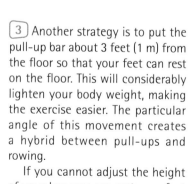

③

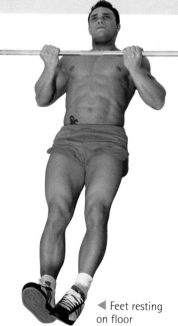

③ Another strategy is to put the pull-up bar about 3 feet (1 m) from the floor so that your feet can rest on the floor. This will considerably lighten your body weight, making the exercise easier. The particular angle of this movement creates a hybrid between pull-ups and rowing.

If you cannot adjust the height of your bar, you can rest your feet on a chair instead.

◄ Feet resting on floor

/// Row

This is a multijoint exercise for the back muscles and the biceps. Unilateral work is very popular for this exercise because it greatly increases the range of motion.

Torso inclined to 120 degrees ▼

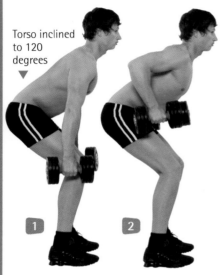

1 Lean forward so that your torso forms a 90- to 120-degree angle to the floor. Hold two dumbbells in a neutral grip (thumbs forward).

2 Pull the arms along the length of the body, bending them so that you raise your elbows as high as possible. Maintain the contracted position for one to two seconds while squeezing your shoulder blades together before you lower the weights.

! The bilateral version of this exercise has some risks for the back, especially when using heavy weights. ● One way to reduce these risks is to avoid bending to 90 degrees. You can lift your torso up a little so that it is only at a 120-degree angle to the floor. It is often easier to feel the muscles work this way. In addition, this position is less dangerous and you will feel stronger using it.

(**Variations**)

1 **2** To do this exercise unilaterally, use your free hand to push against your thigh or a chair so that you support your lower back. Take advantage of the fact that the muscle stretch, and especially the contraction, is much better when you work unilaterally than when you work bilaterally. Try to exaggerate the range of motion when working only one arm at a time.

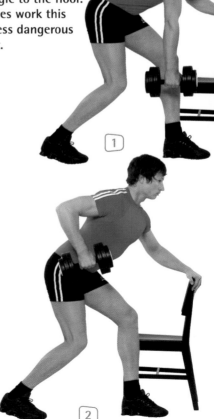

HELPFUL HINTS

As a general rule, you should pull the dumbbells up to your navel. Some people like to bring the weights higher toward the chest and others a little lower, near the thighs. In the same way, with hand positions, some people prefer to have their thumbs slightly turned in and others like them slightly turned out. Choose whichever position is best for your muscles.

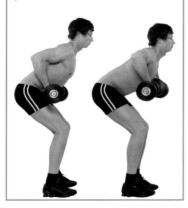

ADVANTAGES

The row mostly works the muscles at the interior of the back, particularly the lower trapezius (see page 139). It will not increase the size of your back as pull-ups will. This is why people say rowing works the thickness of the back. So rowing and pull-ups are complementary exercises for the latissimus dorsi muscles.

- - - - - - - - - - - - - - - - - - - -

The forward-leaning position is not good for intense work because it can interfere with breathing. This precarious position is not very good for the spine, either.

DISADVANTAGES

BACK

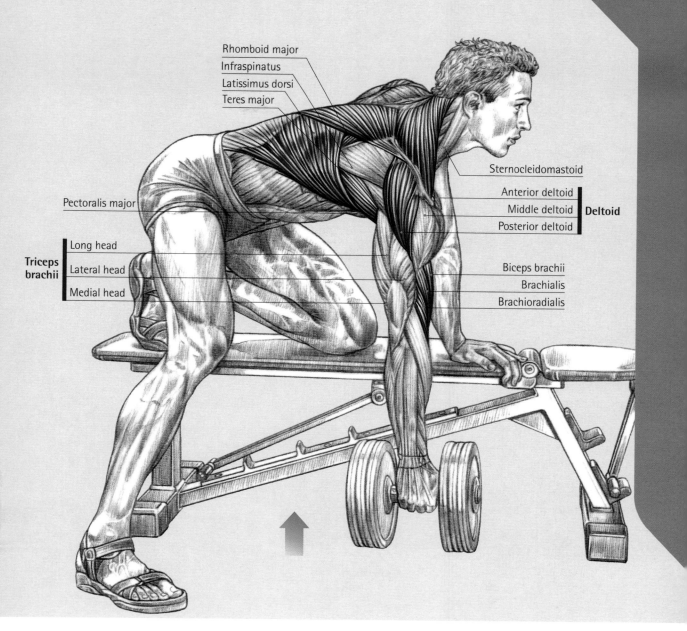

Rhomboid major
Infraspinatus
Latissimus dorsi
Teres major

Sternocleidomastoid

Anterior deltoid
Middle deltoid **Deltoid**
Posterior deltoid

Pectoralis major

Triceps brachii
Long head
Lateral head
Medial head

Biceps brachii
Brachialis
Brachioradialis

③ Bands can be used to great advantage in rowing. Attach one end of a band to your dumbbell and step on the other end.

You can also do the seated row using a band. Put one end of the loop around your feet and hold the other end in your hands (supinated or pronated grip). Using your back muscles, pull your hands to your torso.

NOTES
Keep your head very straight, especially during the contraction phase of the exercise. Avoid turning your head from left to right as people are often tempted to do.

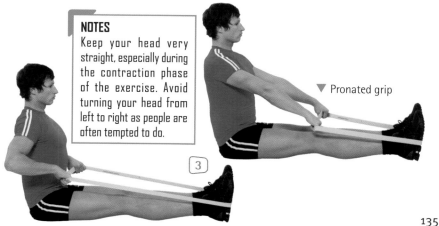

▼ Pronated grip

③

135

/// Bent-Arm Pullover

This is an isolation exercise for the latissimus dorsi muscles and, to a lesser extent, the pectoralis and triceps muscles. It can be done unilaterally in a slightly modified version, which we will explain in detail.

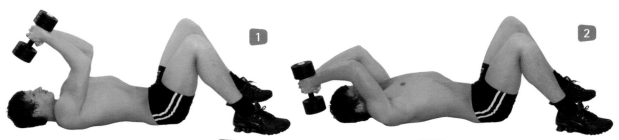

1 Lie down with your back on a bed and your head at the edge of the mattress so that your arms can hang freely when held behind your head. This gives you a greater range of motion and a better stretch than if you did the exercise lying on the floor. Hold a dumbbell with both hands in a neutral grip (thumbs toward the floor) or a pronated grip (thumbs touching), and move your arms (bent to 90 degrees) above your head.

2 Keep your arms bent and lower them behind your head. When your arms are as low as possible, bring them back up using the strength of your latissimus dorsi muscles. Stop the movement when the dumbbell is above your forehead, and then lower the weight again.

▲ Neutral grip

HELPFUL HINTS

This is an exercise that works the latissimus dorsi muscles through stretching, so you must try to go down as low as possible without forcing your shoulders. To maintain continuous tension, do not bring the dumbbell up too high (unless you need to rest at the end of a set so that you can do a few more repetitions).

BACK

Variations

If you cannot feel the latissimus dorsi muscles working well during the classic exercise, there is a unilateral version of this exercise. Instead of lying on your back, lie on your left side.

1 With the right hand in a neutral position (thumb at bottom), move your arm above your head.

2 Go as far forward as possible. Unlike the bilateral pullover, you should always keep your arm straight. So that you can maintain continuous tension, do not bring the dumbbell too high. Once you have finished a set with your right arm, move immediately to your left arm.

This is more of a motor learning exercise than a muscle mass movement. The goal is to constantly feel your latissimus dorsi working. In this way you will learn to feel the contraction of this muscle. Little by little, this sensation of a good contraction will be transferred to other back exercises where you could not feel this muscle working before.

TIP

In the unilateral version, put your free hand on the latissimus dorsi muscle that is working. This strategy will help you to feel the muscle contract better.

NOTES

You can use the pullover to open up the rib cage. However, some stretching exercises are better for expanding the rib cage (see the section on the chest).

136

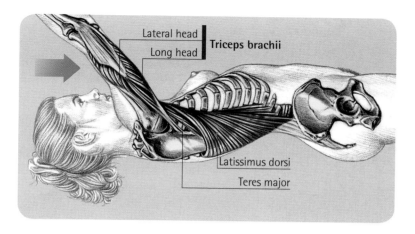

Lateral head

Long head

Triceps brachii

Latissimus dorsi

Teres major

! Pullovers place the shoulder joints in a relatively unstable position. This means you must not use too heavy a weight. You should increase the number of repetitions rather than the weight. Try to feel the muscles more than you feel the performance. Be sure that the weights are securely attached to the bar because you do not want them to fall off when the dumbbell is above your head!

/// Stretching the Back

These two exercises stretch different parts of the back. They are complementary and must be done together rather than you choosing one over the other.

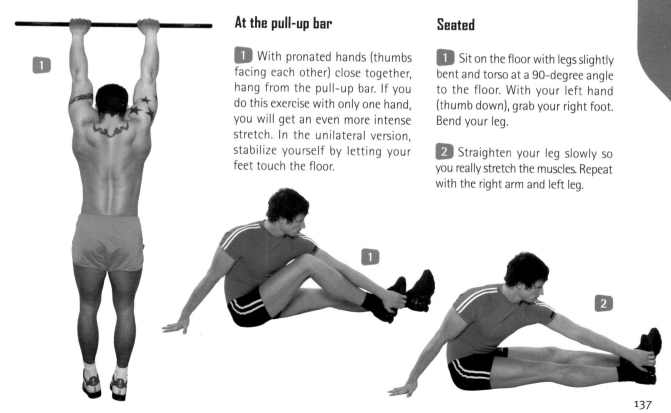

At the pull-up bar

1 With pronated hands (thumbs facing each other) close together, hang from the pull-up bar. If you do this exercise with only one hand, you will get an even more intense stretch. In the unilateral version, stabilize yourself by letting your feet touch the floor.

Seated

1 Sit on the floor with legs slightly bent and torso at a 90-degree angle to the floor. With your left hand (thumb down), grab your right foot. Bend your leg.

2 Straighten your leg slowly so you really stretch the muscles. Repeat with the right arm and left leg.

137

Trapezius

▌Role of the Trapezius

The trapezius muscles are divided into two major parts:

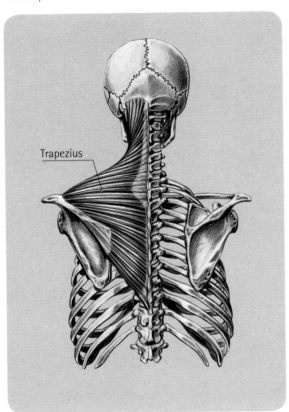

Trapezius

1. Upper-trapezius muscles. These muscles raise the shoulders. The upper-trapezius muscles are useful in contact sports, combat sports, and shot put. Other than the strength they provide, they also protect the neck. Aesthetically, the trapezius muscles create an impressive look that can be seen even though clothing. A large neck and impressive trapezius muscles are ideal for frightening an opponent. This is a classic combination in ultimate fighting and in boxing.

When you do shoulder shrugs, it is usually the upper trapezius that does the work. This is the part we focus on here. Another exercise for the trapezius is the upright row (as described in the shoulder section) using a close grip.

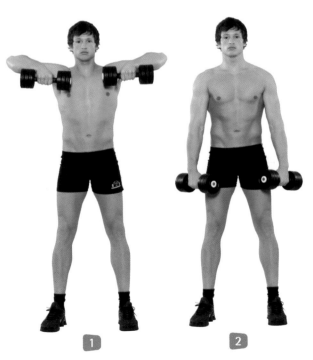

1 2

Action of the trapezius muscles

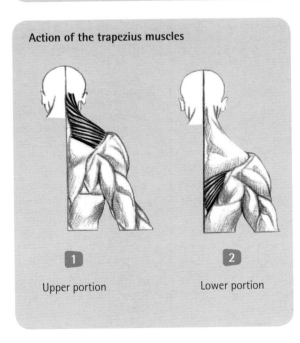

1 2

Upper portion   Lower portion

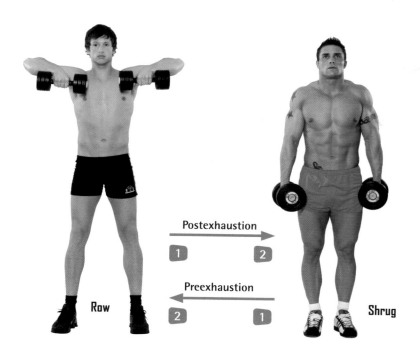

Supersets for the upper trapezius

A **postexhaustion superset** begins with the upright row, dumbbells touching each other. At failure, go immediately to shrugs.

A **preexhaustion superset** begins with shrugs just before the upright row.

Postexhaustion

1 → 2

Preexhaustion

2 ← 1

Row   Shrug

2. Lower-trapezius muscles. These muscles perform the opposite task of the upper-trapezius muscles by lowering the arms. They are antagonistic to the upper trapezius, and they also bring the shoulder blades together. For athletes, the purpose of the lower trapezius is, above all, to stabilize, and therefore protect, the shoulder joint. A weak lower-trapezius muscle encourages deltoid injuries. For this reason, it is much more important to develop the lower trapezius than the upper trapezius. The primary exercises that work the lower trapezius are rows and lateral raises done while leaning forward.

Row

Postexhaustion

1 → 2

Preexhaustion

2 ← 1

Lateral raise

Supersets for the lower trapezius

A **postexhaustion superset** begins with rowing. At failure, go immediately to lateral raises.

A **preexhaustion superset** begins with lateral raises just before rowing.

! Scientific studies show a large disparity in development between the upper and lower trapezius in strong athletes. When athletes are compared with sedentary people who have the same body weight, the athletes have much stronger upper-trapezius muscles than sedentary people. However, in the lower trapezius, athletes are no stronger than sedentary people. This is an imbalance that will negatively affect performance. You should correct this common imbalance as soon as possible by doing more rowing and more lateral raises for the back.

/// Shrug

This is an isolation exercise for the upper trapezius.
Unilateral work is possible but not desirable.

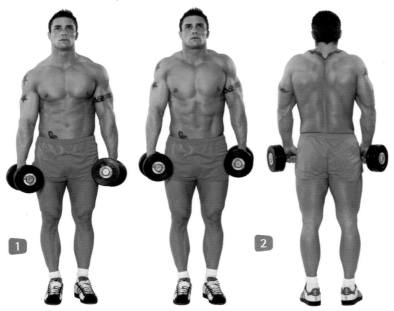

! Because of their proximity to the cervical spine, repeated contractions of the upper-trapezius muscles can cause headaches ranging from mild pain to migraines. You should therefore introduce this exercise slowly during workouts and increase your weight progressively.

1 Stand with your arms by your sides. Grab two dumbbells using a neutral grip (thumbs forward).

2 Bring your shoulders up as if you were trying to touch your ears. When your shoulders are as high as they can go, hold the contracted position for one second. Then lower your shoulders as much as you can.

HELPFUL HINTS
Do not bend the arms at the beginning of the movement. However, at the end of the movement, you can pull lightly with your biceps in order to raise your shoulders just a bit higher.

NOTES
Incidentally, if it does not bother you, it is best to begin your chest or shoulder workout with a little trapezius work. This will help you warm up the shoulder joints and wake up the central nervous system. But this warm-up should not interfere with the rest of your workout. For example, you should not have trouble with other exercises because your trapezius muscles are on fire.

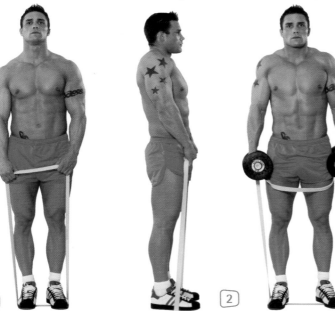

Variations

1 **2** A band held under your feet can replace the dumbbells or can be used in addition to the dumbbells.

3 You can put the dumbbells in front of or behind your body to change the angle of attack on the trapezius muscles.

BACK

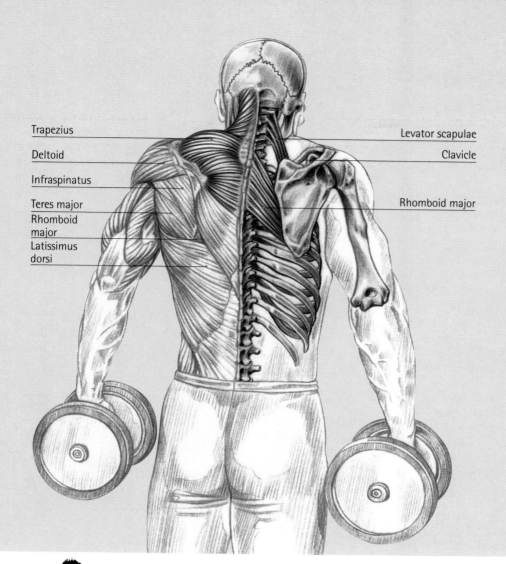

Trapezius

Deltoid

Infraspinatus

Teres major

Rhomboid major

Latissimus dorsi

Levator scapulae

Clavicle

Rhomboid major

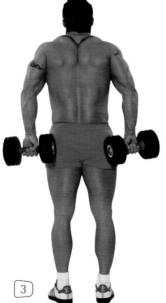

3

The following combination can tire out the trapezius in minimal time. Begin the shrug exercise with your arms slightly behind you and with hands in a pronated grip (thumbs facing each other). At failure, bring them to the sides (neutral grip) so you can continue the exercise using an easier version. When you reach failure again, pull your arms in front (hands in pronated grip) and do a few more repetitions by cheating a little. You should quickly feel an intense burn throughout the upper-trapezius muscles.

ADVANTAGES

This exercise works directly on the trapezius without interference from other small muscles that could tire out before the trapezius.

The upper trapezius is easy to develop. The lower trapezius is more difficult to strengthen, and it is often neglected. This creates an imbalance between antagonistic muscles. Rather than continually working the upper trapezius, it is better to spend more time working the lower trapezius.

DISADVANTAGES

Lumbar Muscles

▌Role of the Lumbar Muscles

Lumbar muscles have two purposes:

1 As their name indicates, these back muscles support the lower part of the spine. When they are sufficiently developed, these muscles will handle any pressure applied to the lower back instead of the spine. This is why they are useful in almost all sports. For those who are only weight training, solid lumbar muscles will allow you to perform multijoint exercises without danger because, in general, these exercises have a tendency to compress the spine.

2 Lumbar muscles are also responsible for bringing the torso upright from a forward-leaning position. In this task, the lumbar muscles rarely work alone; they typically work at the same time as the glutes and the hamstrings.

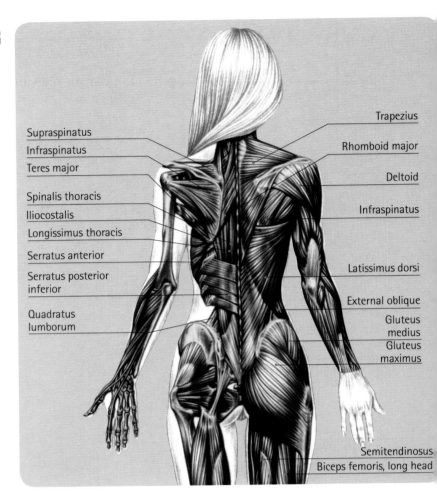

Supraspinatus
Infraspinatus
Teres major
Spinalis thoracis
Iliocostalis
Longissimus thoracis
Serratus anterior
Serratus posterior inferior
Quadratus lumborum
Trapezius
Rhomboid major
Deltoid
Infraspinatus
Latissimus dorsi
External oblique
Gluteus medius
Gluteus maximus
Semitendinosus
Biceps femoris, long head

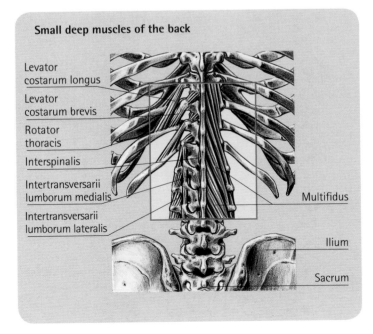

Small deep muscles of the back

Levator costarum longus
Levator costarum brevis
Rotator thoracis
Interspinalis
Intertransversarii lumborum medialis
Intertransversarii lumborum lateralis
Multifidus
Ilium
Sacrum

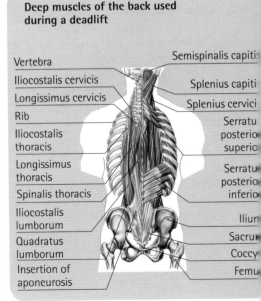

Deep muscles of the back used during a deadlift

Vertebra
Iliocostalis cervicis
Longissimus cervicis
Rib
Iliocostalis thoracis
Longissimus thoracis
Spinalis thoracis
Iliocostalis lumborum
Quadratus lumborum
Insertion of aponeurosis
Semispinalis capitis
Splenius capiti
Splenius cervici
Serratu posterio superio
Serratu posterio inferio
Iliu
Sacru
Coccy
Femu

BACK

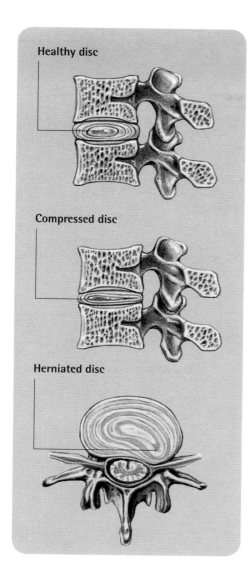

Healthy disc

Compressed disc

Herniated disc

! In weight training, it is easier to hurt your back than it is to strengthen it. Even a small backache will prevent you from training in the gym as well as in your sport. It is imperative that you pay attention to your spine. It is very fragile! It was not made to support the heavy weights required by intense athletic training. To shift the pressure from the spine to the lumbar muscles, you need both strong lumbar muscles and solid abdominal muscles. Just as for the neck muscles, it is important not to injure your back while you are trying to strengthen it!

/// Bent-Legged Deadlift

This is a multijoint exercise not only for the lumbar muscles but also the latissimus dorsi, glutes, and thighs. It can be done unilaterally on one leg.

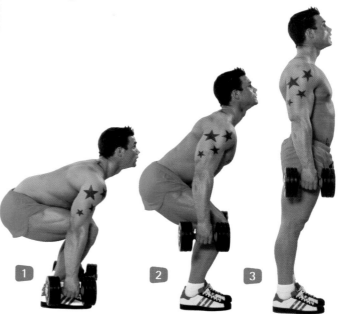

1 With your feet shoulder-width apart, bend over and pick up two dumbbells that you have placed on the floor next to your feet. Keep your back flat and very slightly arched. Use whatever hand grip feels natural. Ideally, you should use a semipronated grip, somewhere between a neutral grip (thumbs forward) and a pronated grip (thumbs facing each other).

2 Push on your legs and pull with your back to stand up. The movements of the legs and back should be synchronized as much as possible. You should not push with your legs first and then pull with your back.

3 Once you are standing up, lean forward while bending your legs to return to your starting position.

143

HELPFUL HINTS

When the lumbar muscles get tired, it becomes more and more difficult to maintain the slight natural arch of the back. The spine will start to curve. This arch in the back makes the exercise easier and will help you do a few more repetitions. That is why very few people stop the exercise when they feel the arch in their back change.

However, continuing the exercise when the lumbar discs are in a bad position due to fatigue is not a good idea. It is better to stop the exercise when you feel your back begin to curve. If you want to continue the exercise, lighten the weight. For example, you can use only one dumbbell placed between your legs and held in both hands.

NOTES

You might feel that you have to go too low to pick the weights up off the floor, especially if you have longer legs and short arms. You will then have to curve your back to grab the weights, which is a bad movement for your back. In this case, you should set the weights on large phone books to reduce the range of motion.

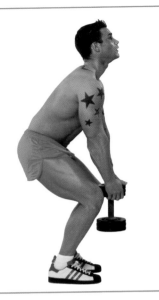

! This exercise works the spine intensely. There is a serious risk of compressing the intervertebral discs, especially if your back is in a bad position. As at the end of every workout, particularly those where you have worked the lumbar region, you should stretch for a long time at the pull-up bar.

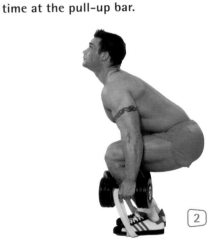

1

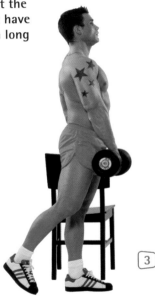

2

3

BACK

Variations

1 Instead of using weights, you can use a band. Stand on the band and grab one end in each hand.

2 You can also combine a band with dumbbells for maximum effectiveness. In fact, dumbbells mostly provide resistance at the beginning of the exercise and much less at the end. The band has the opposite effect. Combining the two will provide resistance throughout the exercise.

3 You can also do the exercise while standing on one leg.

144

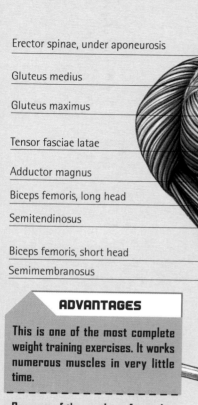

Erector spinae, under aponeurosis

Gluteus medius

Gluteus maximus

Tensor fasciae latae

Adductor magnus

Biceps femoris, long head

Semitendinosus

Biceps femoris, short head

Semimembranosus

/// Stretching the Spinal Column

To decompress your spine, hang from the pull-up bar, as described on page 37.

However, we do not advise you to stretch your lumbar muscles using exercises that require bending for-ward (either sitting or standing) when you have just done exercises that compromise your interverte-bral discs. Reserve the following stretches for another day.

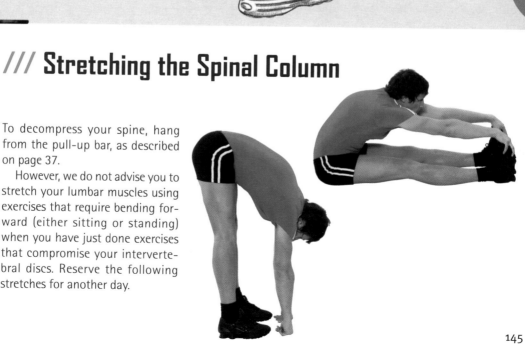

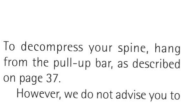

/// Clean and Jerk Dumbbell Lift

This is a multijoint exercise for the lumbar region, latissimus dorsi, glutes, thighs, and arms.
The shoulders also work very hard in the version where you lift your arms above your head. This latter version is what weightlifters call the clean and jerk, which is the most complete weight training movement because almost all of the muscles in the body take part. Unilateral work is not a good idea.

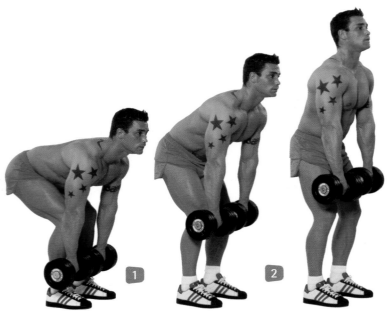 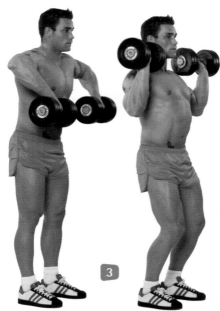

1 Bend over so you can pick up two dumbbells that are on the floor next to your feet. Keep your back flat and very slightly arched. Use a natural hand grip; semipronated would be ideal.

2 Push with your legs and pull with your back to stand up. The leg and back movements should be synchronized as much as possible.

3 Once you are almost standing up, use your momentum to bend your arms (hands almost pronated) and bring the weights to your shoulders.

COMMENT
When we mention the partial clean and jerk, this means that the exercise stops when the dumbbells reach shoulder level. The complete clean and jerk refers to the exercise when it is done with the full range of motion (that is, with the arms straight above the head).

HELPFUL HINTS
Be sure to warm up very well before using heavy weights. Your warm-up should not only prepare your muscles but also condition you to the technical execution of the exercise.

NOTES
Keep your head very straight and your gaze slightly up. Most important, avoid looking left or right because this can cause an imbalance and result in a back injury.

This is an explosive movement, so it is potentially dangerous. Attempt this exercise with extreme caution. Do not begin immediately with heavy weights.

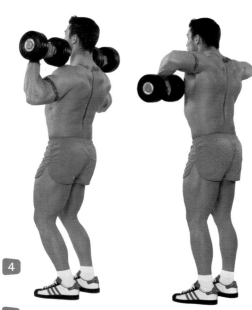

4

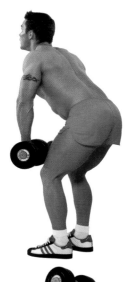

4 From there, lower the dumbbells and lean forward while bending your legs to return to the starting position.

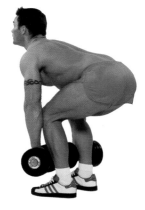

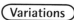

ADVANTAGES

The clean and jerk lift works several muscle groups in a short time. Not only does it exercise the muscles, but it also helps improve your motor coordination. In long sets, it is also excellent for increasing strength and endurance.

- -

This is a very technical exercise that requires a certain amount of time to learn as well as to gain muscle mastery. Even though it helps athletes enormously, we do not advise this exercise for people who have fewer than two months of weight training experience.

DISADVANTAGES

Variations

v Alternatively, for a more complete exercise that is less focused on the back, you can straighten your arms above your head to do the lift using the full range of motion.

147

STRENGTHEN YOUR THIGHS

Quadriceps

▌Role of the Quadriceps

Generally, when playing sports, the thighs are used much more often than the muscles in the torso. Thigh muscles help you run and jump, two indispensable elements in numerous sports. Medical research has clearly demonstrated the direct relationship between muscle mass in the thighs and their capacity to generate power during a sprint on foot or on a bicycle. In other words, the more muscular your quadriceps are, the faster you can go. A woman who has thighs that are as muscular as a man's can run practically as fast as he can. Thus, we can see the importance of training the lower part of the body to improve performance when speed is required.

Aesthetically, large thighs are much less desirable than a muscular torso. The thighs are often neglected. However, they should be well developed, and you can develop them quickly using the following exercises.

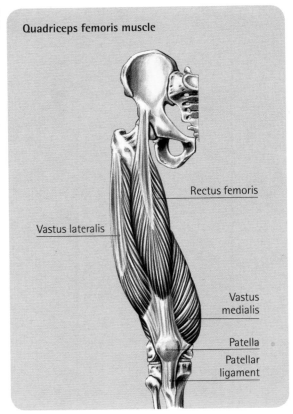

Quadriceps femoris muscle

Rectus femoris

Vastus lateralis

Vastus medialis

Patella

Patellar ligament

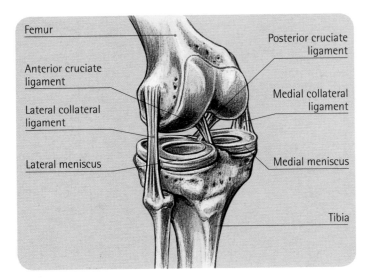

Femur

Anterior cruciate ligament

Lateral collateral ligament

Lateral meniscus

Posterior cruciate ligament

Medial collateral ligament

Medial meniscus

Tibia

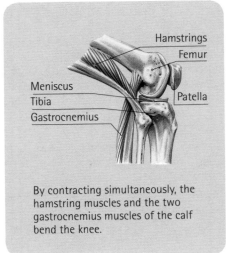

Hamstrings

Femur

Meniscus

Tibia

Gastrocnemius

Patella

By contracting simultaneously, the hamstring muscles and the two gastrocnemius muscles of the calf bend the knee.

! Before working the thighs, protect the knees by warming up all the muscles that attach to the knees. Too often, a knee warm-up consists simply of warming up the quadriceps. This is a mistake! To avoid knee problems, you must begin by warming up the hamstrings, then the quadriceps, and finally the calves. Many small aches and pains will be eliminated or prevented if you follow this simple rule.

/// Squat

This is a multijoint exercise for the quadriceps, hamstrings, lumbar muscles, calves, and glutes. Although you can do this exercise unilaterally on one leg, we do not recommend it.

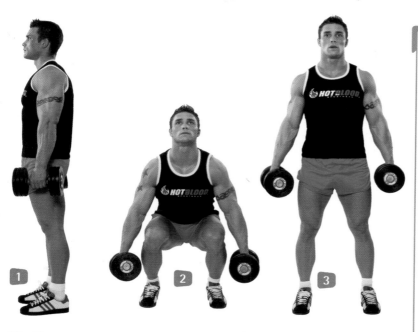

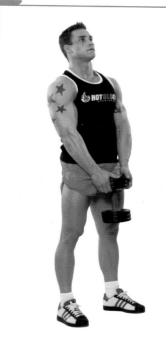

1 2 With your feet about shoulder-width apart, bend over so you can pick up two dumbbells on the floor. Keep your back flat and very slightly arched backward. Use a neutral hand grip (thumbs forward). The ideal would be to use a semipronated grip—a grip somewhere between a neutral grip and a pronated grip (thumbs facing each other).

3 Keeping the back as straight as possible, push on your legs until they are straight. Once you are upright, bend your legs and return to the starting position. Do not go all the way to the floor, but only just until you feel that you are starting to really bend forward at the waist. At the moment when you have to bend forward too much, the work on the thighs diminishes and the lumbar muscles begin to do the majority of the work.

HELPFUL HINTS

The farther you go down, the more you will pull your heels off the floor to keep your back straight. With your heels unstable, the work is done by the quadriceps. On the contrary, if you keep your heels on the floor, you will have a harder time keeping your back straight. Then your glutes, hamstrings, and lumbar muscles will do more of the work.

When you reach failure, if you want to continue the exercise, lighten the weight by using only one dumbbell placed between your legs and held with both of your hands. After that, you can lay this dumbbell aside and do the exercise with no weight.

Variations

There are many variations of the squat:

Variation in the Level of Descent
The lower you go, the more difficult the squat becomes since it recruits a growing number of muscle groups. However, the level of descent must take into account not only the muscles that you want to focus on but also your anatomy. The longer your legs are, particularly your thighs, the more dangerous it is for the back if you go very low. An unfavorable leg-to-torso ratio will mean that you lean very far forward and make the lumbar muscles unstable.

Inclination of the torso in the squat according to different morphologies

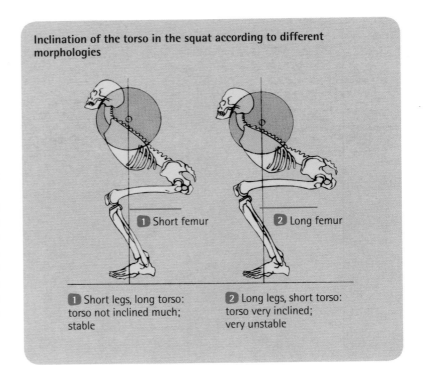

1 Short femur   2 Long femur

1 Short legs, long torso: torso not inclined much; stable

2 Long legs, short torso: torso very inclined; very unstable

Box Squat
To define the range of how low to go, use a bed or a chair. This exercise is not about landing heavily on the bed or the chair so that you stop. The box squat should be done in a controlled manner so that you land softly. From here, there are two possible variations:

1 As soon as you land, come immediately back up without stopping. This modified plyometric exercise promotes muscle explosiveness.

2 Sit down for one to two seconds to relax your muscles. This stop-and-go technique improves your starting strength, which is indispensable for athletes who must do sprints from a stopped position.

NOTE
Some people do not like the box squat at all. Other people can feel their thighs working only if there is something stopping them and defining the length of descent. Do not fight nature! Choose the version that allows you to feel your thighs working the most.

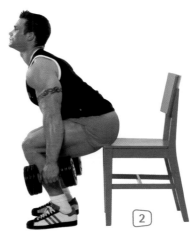

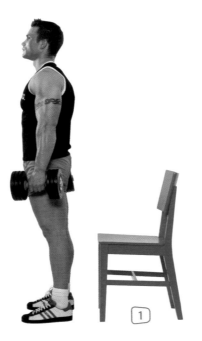

1

2

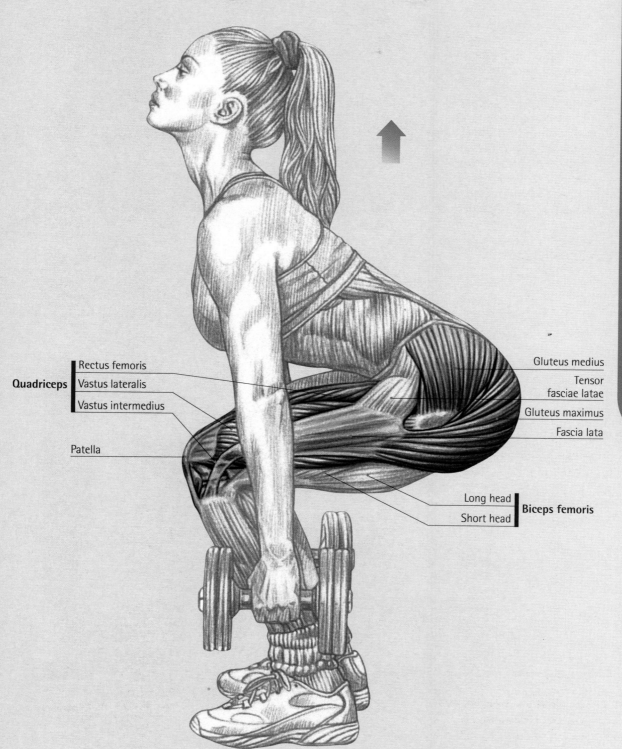

Quadriceps
- Rectus femoris
- Vastus lateralis
- Vastus intermedius

Patella

Gluteus medius

Tensor
fasciae latae

Gluteus maximus

Fascia lata

Long head

Short head

Biceps femoris

Width of the Feet

[v] It is possible to vary the width of your feet. It is better to keep them about shoulder width and slightly turned out so that the entire thigh does equal work. To focus the work on the quadriceps, make your stance narrower, even very narrow. In this case, the knees are much more involved. You can also use a very wide stance, which will make the inner thighs, hamstrings, and glutes work more. As with all variations, at first you should choose the one that feels most natural to you. Later, you can progressively adopt a position that targets the zones that you wish to work.

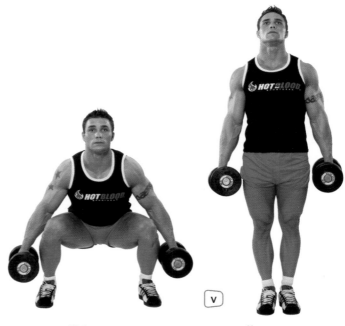

Wide squat   [v]   Narrow squat

Continuous Tension

[1] [2] The more you straighten your legs, the more you lose muscular tension, because the exercise becomes easier at the top of the movement. To remedy this problem, you can step on a band and hold the ends in your hands. In this case, the more you straighten the legs, the more resistance is created, which responds perfectly to the way strength works in the thighs.

[3] Ideally, you could combine dumbbells and a band.

Another solution is to never fully straighten the legs at the top of the movement so that you maintain continuous tension. The exercise becomes much more difficult because the muscles can no longer rest at the top of the squat. You can begin the exercise without straightening the legs. At failure, straighten them so that you can rest a little and do a few more repetitions.

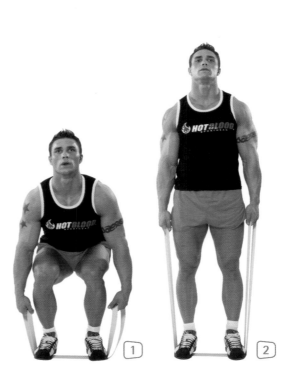

Squat with band   Squat with band plus dumbbells

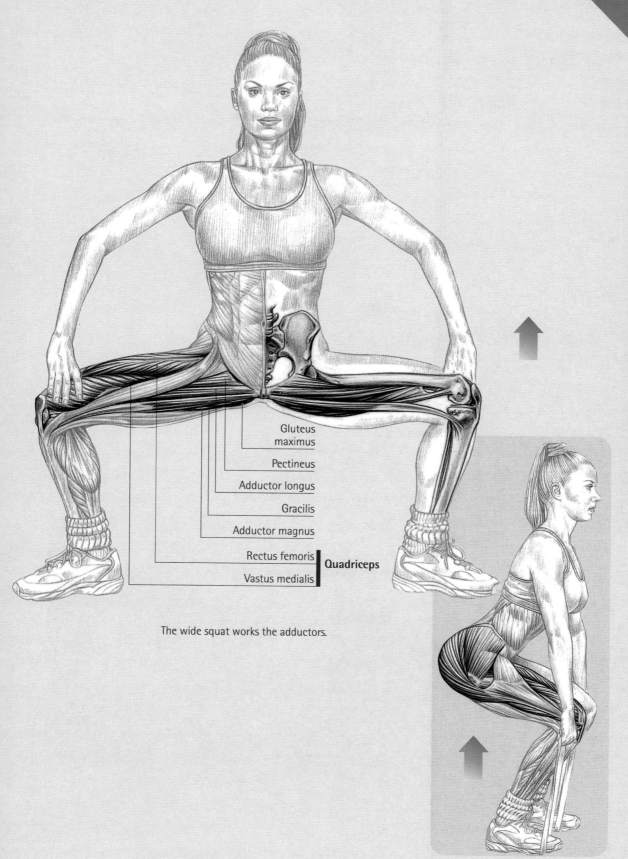

Gluteus
maximus

Pectineus

Adductor longus

Gracilis

Adductor magnus

Rectus femoris | **Quadriceps**

Vastus medialis

The wide squat works the adductors.

/// Unilateral Squat

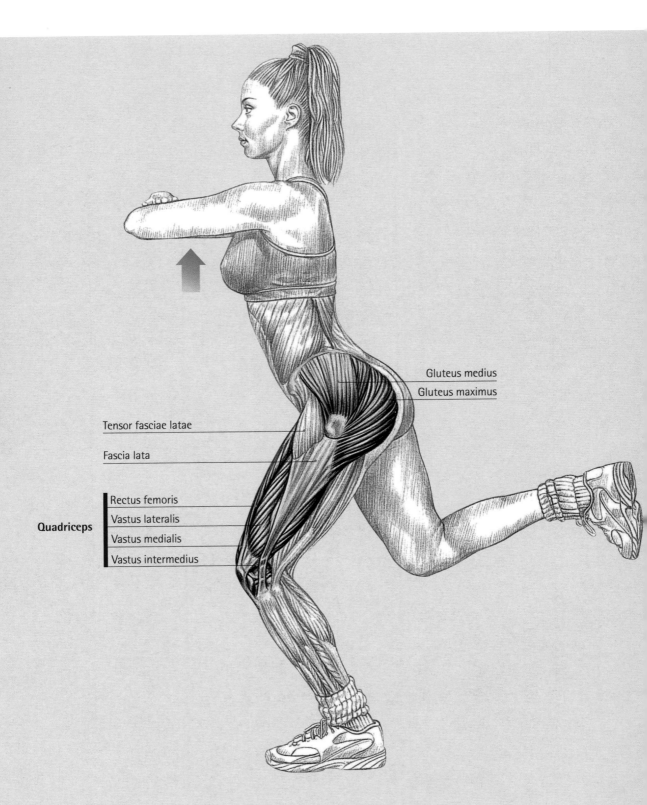

Gluteus medius

Gluteus maximus

Tensor fasciae latae

Fascia lata

Quadriceps
- Rectus femoris
- Vastus lateralis
- Vastus medialis
- Vastus intermedius

LEGS

154

/// Squat and Lift

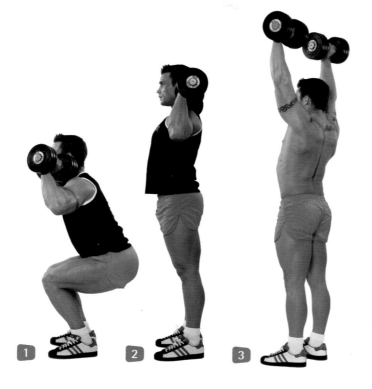

1 2 3

ADVANTAGES

Squats work the entire lower body in a short time. This exercise is harsh (that is, it entails great metabolic stimulation for the growth of the whole body). In fact, more than any other movement, squats trigger the natural secretion of anabolic hormones (testosterone and growth hormone) when you push to your maximum ability.

This exhausting exercise carries some risk for the back and knees.

DISADVANTAGES

! The knees, hips, and spine are heavily used during squats. Do not work against nature by trying to go lower than your body type will allow. Some people are made to go low and others are not! Respect your joints or they will make you pay for it later. It is smarter not to go too low than to go too low.

Just as at the end of every workout where you have worked your lumbar muscles, you should stretch for a long time at the pull-up bar.

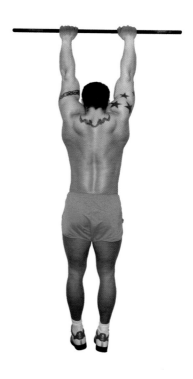

/// Sissy Squat

This is an isolation exercise especially for the quadriceps. It can be done unilaterally. The sissy squat is very different from a classic squat. With it you can work without weights, which protects the back and the hips.

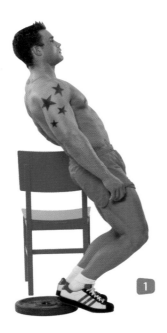

1 To avoid balance problems, hold onto a chair or a wall. Your feet should be about shoulder-width apart. Lean backward while bending and moving your knees forward. The lower you go, the more you need to glue your heels to the floor. Keep your back very straight without arching it. First go down a few inches before coming back up. If you do not come all the way up, you can keep your legs from straightening and maintain continuous tension in the quadriceps. Go lower and lower with each repetition.

HELPFUL HINTS

Putting a wedge beneath your heels makes this exercise easier to do. The higher the wedge, the easier the movement will be. Beginners should start doing this exercise with a wedge. Later, once you are comfortable with the exercise, remove the wedge.

NOTES

This exercise is done slowly and under continuous tension. It is not an exercise done explosively with heavy weights. It is often used during physical therapy for the patellar ligament (see page 255).

ADVANTAGES

The sissy squat requires a lot of work from the central part of the quadriceps. It is the only head in the quadriceps that is multijoint. This part of the muscle, often neglected, is very important for athletes who run or jump.

- - - - - - - - - - - - - - - - - - - -

The knees must be really warm before starting this exercise. Ideally, this should not be the first thigh exercise of your workout.

DISADVANTAGES

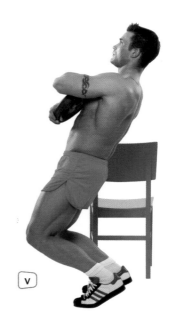

(**Variations**)

v To add resistance, you can hold a weight plate against your chest with one or both hands.

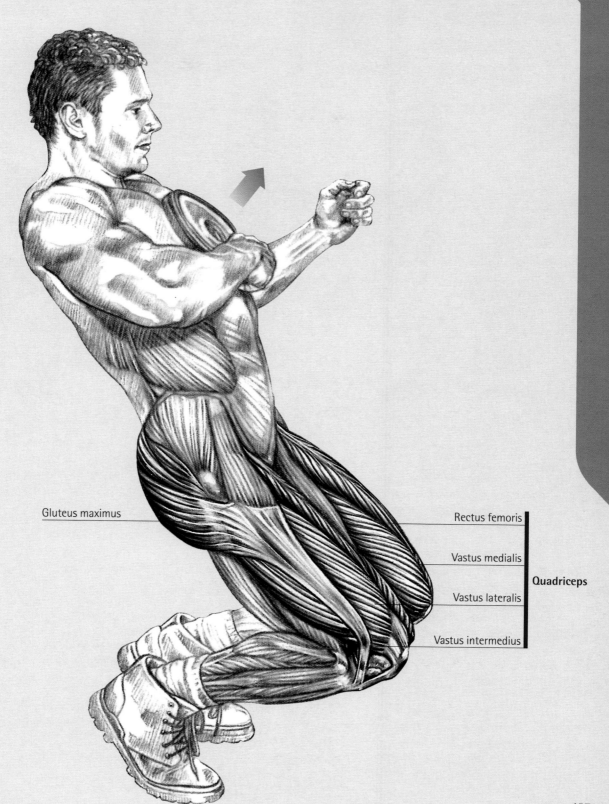

Gluteus maximus

Rectus femoris

Vastus medialis

Quadriceps

Vastus lateralis

Vastus intermedius

/// Leg Lift

This is a multijoint exercise especially for the rectus femoris, abdominals, and psoas major.
This exercise must be done unilaterally. This is a great exercise for sprinters and jumpers.

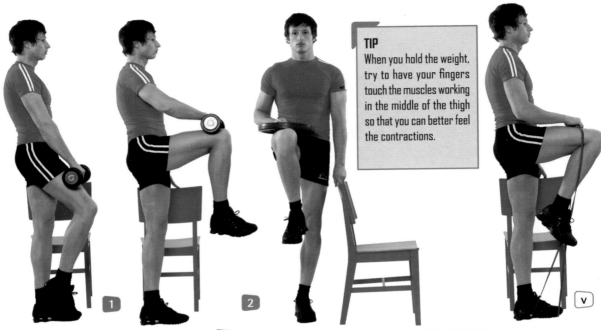

TIP
When you hold the weight, try to have your fingers touch the muscles working in the middle of the thigh so that you can better feel the contractions.

1 Stand up and put a weight plate or a dumbbell on your right thigh, a little above the knee. Stabilize the weight with your right hand while the left hand holds onto the back of a chair or a wall to provide stability. You can also put your back against a wall.

2 Lift the leg until it is parallel to the floor by bending the knee. Hold the contraction for one second before lowering the thigh until it is perpendicular to the floor.

Variations

v With the hand holding the weight, you can push on the thigh while lowering it to accentuate the negative phase of the movement. When the thigh is tired, stop the accentuated negatives so that you can do a few additional classic repetitions. At failure, set the weight down so you can continue the exercise. If you can, begin doing the negative pushes again so you end up doing your maximum number of repetitions.

Instead of a dumbbell, you can attach a band above the knee and put the other end under your foot on the floor.

You can also use a band plus a weight to take advantage of the synergy provided by these two types of resistance.

! **Working the psoas major pulls on your spine. Keep your back very straight and avoid any arching of the low back. If you hear creaking sounds from the spine, then do not lift the leg as high and do the exercise more slowly. If the creaking sounds persist, then do not perform this exercise.**

HELPFUL HINTS
Do not touch your foot to the floor between each repetition. By not moving the thigh all the way down, you maintain continuous tension. Only at failure should you rest the foot on the floor to breathe for a second and then do a few additional repetitions.

NOTES
If you have difficulty warming up your quadriceps before working your thighs, a few sets of leg lifts can help you. Moreover, if your knees prevent you from really working your quadriceps, then this exercise will work a part of the muscle without hurting your kneecaps.

LEGS

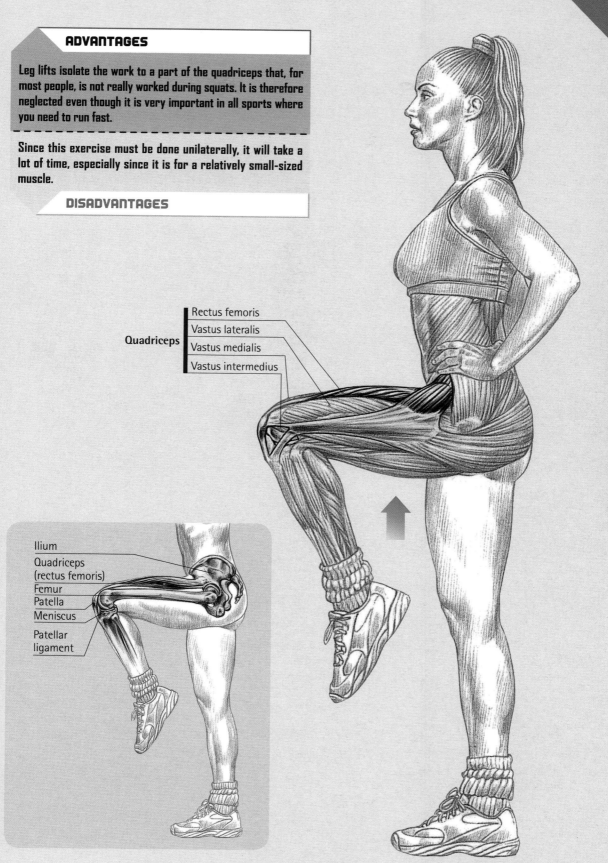

ADVANTAGES

Leg lifts isolate the work to a part of the quadriceps that, for most people, is not really worked during squats. It is therefore neglected even though it is very important in all sports where you need to run fast.

Since this exercise must be done unilaterally, it will take a lot of time, especially since it is for a relatively small-sized muscle.

DISADVANTAGES

Quadriceps
- Rectus femoris
- Vastus lateralis
- Vastus medialis
- Vastus intermedius

Ilium
Quadriceps
(rectus femoris)
Femur
Patella
Meniscus
Patellar
ligament

/// Lunge

This multijoint exercise works the entire thigh. It is similar to a one-legged squat, and it must be done unilaterally.

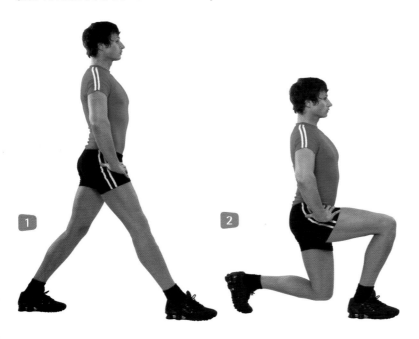

1 Stand with your feet close together and your legs straight. Place your hands on your hips or thighs. If you have balance problems, hold onto a wall or a chair. Begin the exercise by taking a big step forward with your right leg. Beginners can bend the left leg a little bit. Those with more experience can keep the left leg straight to make the exercise harder.

2 Bend the right knee a little bit. Beginners should go down only eight inches or so while others can go as far down as possible. When the knee is bent enough, push with the leg to straighten it again. Start another repetition by bending the knee if you choose to maintain continuous tension. You can also choose to bring the feet back together (see the variations). Repeat the same exercise on the left leg.

! The knees and hips work very hard when you do lunges, but your back is spared.

ADVANTAGES

Lunges allow you to work the entire thigh without compressing the spine. They are also an excellent stretch for all the muscles of the lower body.

- - - - - - - - - - - - - - - -

Since they stretch the psoas major, lunges have a tendency to make you arch your lower back if those muscles are not very flexible. Pay attention to your posture.

The farther the knee advances in relation to the foot, the more the kneecap will have to work.

DISADVANTAGES

TIP
If you have one hand free, rest it on the muscle you want to isolate so that you can better feel the muscle contracting.

LEGS

160

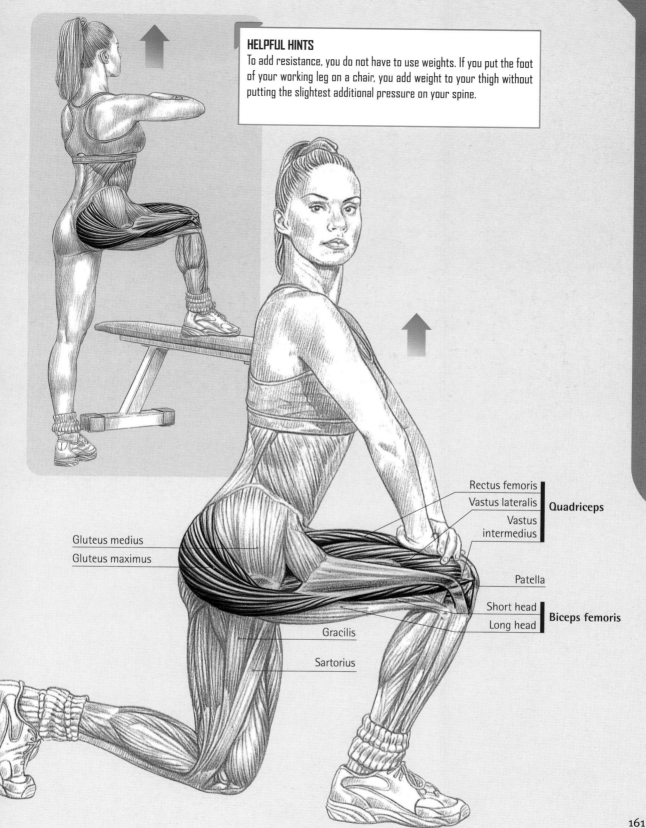

HELPFUL HINTS
To add resistance, you do not have to use weights. If you put the foot of your working leg on a chair, you add weight to your thigh without putting the slightest additional pressure on your spine.

Rectus femoris
Vastus lateralis — **Quadriceps**
Vastus intermedius

Gluteus medius
Gluteus maximus

Patella

Short head — **Biceps femoris**
Long head

Gracilis

Sartorius

161

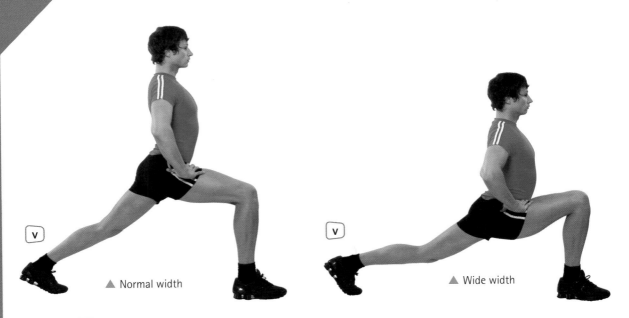

▲ Normal width

▲ Wide width

Variations

There are many variations of lunges.

[v] The first step that you take forward will determine the width of the exercise. It can be narrow or wide. Begin with a small step because it will be easier for you to master the exercise this way. To increase the difficulty, take progressively larger steps.

You can take a step forward or a step backward, depending on your preference.

You can alternate working the left and right leg on every repetition, or you can do an entire set on one leg and then move to the other leg.

You can stand up completely or rest your foot on the floor and do only a partial movement.

> **NOTES**
> The wider the stance you take, the more the glutes and the hamstrings will have to work. It is the same if you lean forward a little. A narrower stance will make the quadriceps work harder.

[1] You can add weight by holding a dumbbell in each hand.

[2] Instead of doing a forward lunge, you can do a side lunge. These lateral lunges are more risky for the knees, but they are closer to the kind of muscle work required in certain sports like soccer or martial arts.

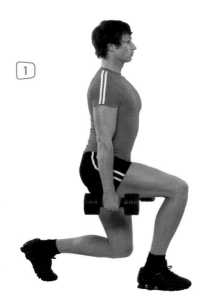

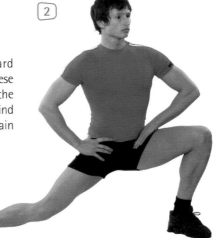

LEGS

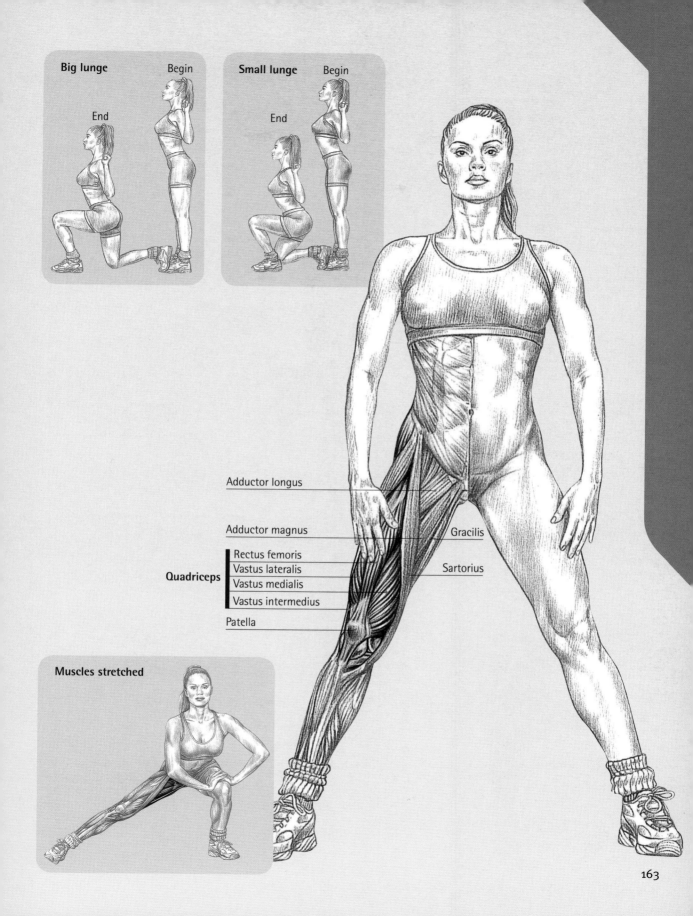

Big lunge   Begin

End

Small lunge   Begin

End

Adductor longus

Adductor magnus

Gracilis

Quadriceps
Rectus femoris
Vastus lateralis
Vastus medialis
Vastus intermedius

Sartorius

Patella

Muscles stretched

163

Adductors

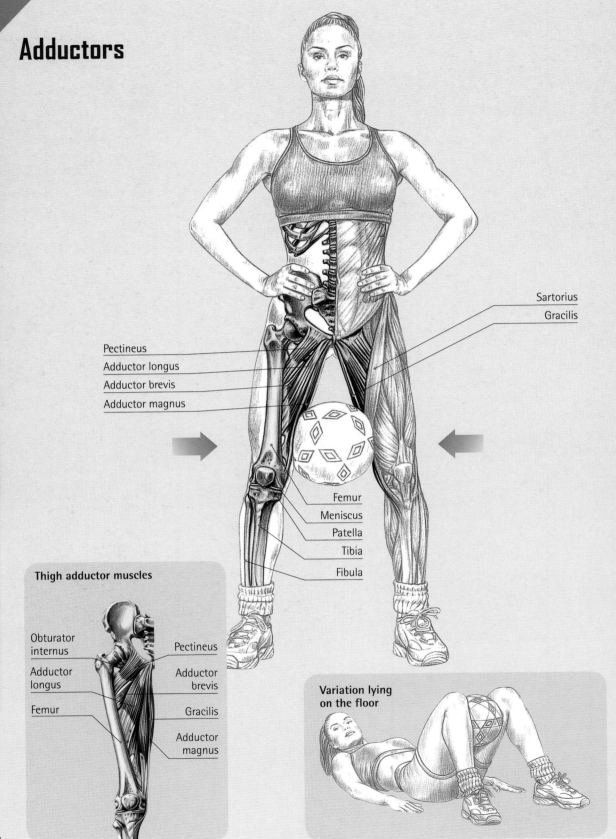

Sartorius

Gracilis

Pectineus

Adductor longus

Adductor brevis

Adductor magnus

Femur

Meniscus

Patella

Tibia

Fibula

LEGS

Thigh adductor muscles

Obturator internus

Pectineus

Adductor longus

Adductor brevis

Femur

Gracilis

Adductor magnus

Variation lying on the floor

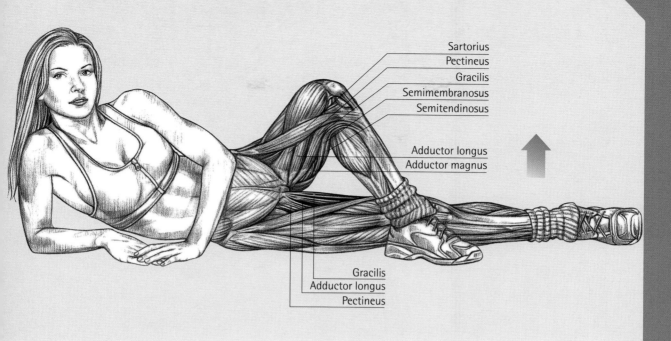

Sartorius
Pectineus
Gracilis
Semimembranosus
Semitendinosus

Adductor longus
Adductor magnus

Gracilis
Adductor longus
Pectineus

1 **2** You can work the adductor muscles of the thighs by squeezing the thighs while working against resistance (such as arm strength, a machine, or a ball).

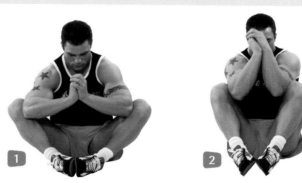

/// Stretching the Adductors

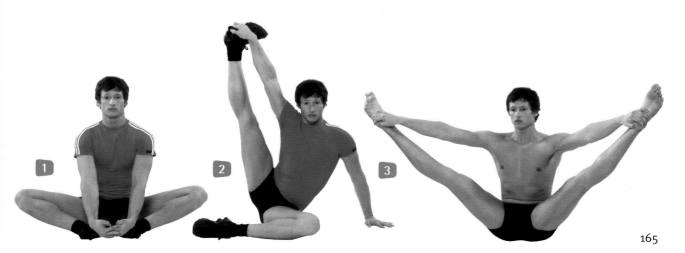

/// Leg Extension

This isolation exercise is the best way to work the quadriceps. Leg extensions can be done unilaterally using a band.

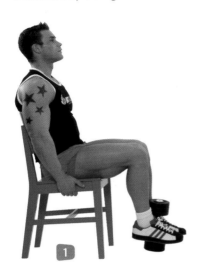

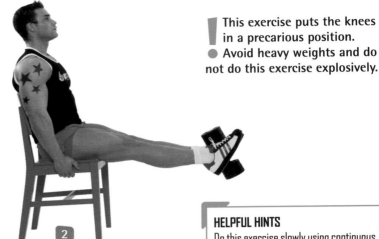

! This exercise puts the knees in a precarious position.
● Avoid heavy weights and do not do this exercise explosively.

1 Sit as far back on a chair as possible so that your feet do not touch the floor. Put a dumbbell between your ankles.

2 Using your quadriceps, straighten your legs. Maintain the contracted position for two to three seconds before lowering.

HELPFUL HINTS
Do this exercise slowly using continuous tension and long sets. It is a good warm-up for the knee. You can also use it as a preexhaustion exercise before squats so that you will really be able to feel your quadriceps working.

NOTES
Leg extensions are either a warm-up exercise or a cool-down exercise for the end of a workout. But you should not count on this exercise to give you massive thighs. However, leg extensions are exceptionally good for defining the quadriceps muscles by reducing fat in that area.

LEGS

Variations

v Instead of holding a dumbbell, you can use a band wrapped around your feet. The other part of the band should be attached behind the chair. Using the band, you can work only one thigh at a time.

Ideally, you could use a band plus a dumbbell to achieve optimal resistance.

ADVANTAGES

The spine does not have to work much in this exercise. The isolation of the quadriceps is almost perfect because the hamstrings are only slightly involved.

This exercise is an artificial movement not found in nature. The quadriceps muscles are meant to work in concert with the hamstrings to provide good protection for the knees. In the absence of active support from the hamstrings, some people's knees may not handle leg extensions well.

DISADVANTAGES

/// Plyometric Exercises for the Thighs

Plyometric exercises for the thighs involve jumping in place.

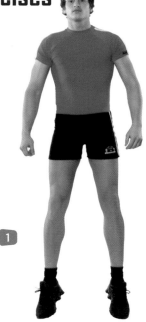

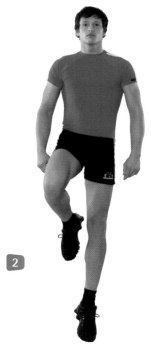

1 In the simplest version, you can jump on both legs at the same time.

2 To increase the difficulty, you can jump on only one leg.

3 You can also jump from a small height for added difficulty.

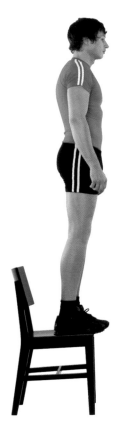

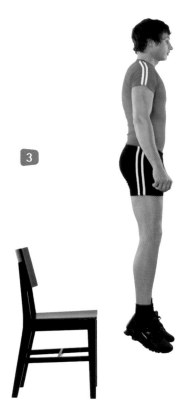

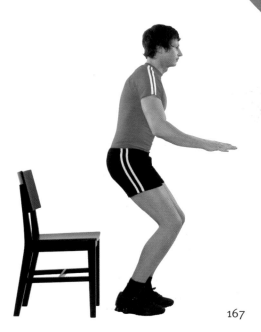

/// Stretching the Quadriceps

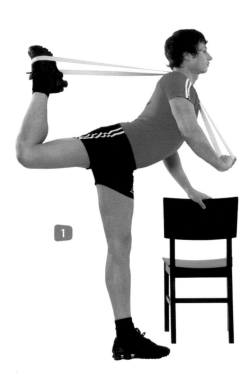

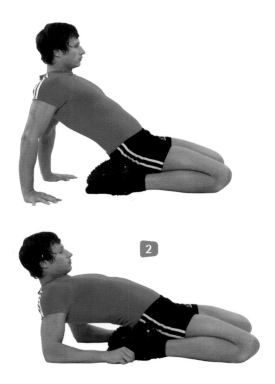

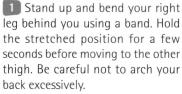

1 Stand up and bend your right leg behind you using a band. Hold the stretched position for a few seconds before moving to the other thigh. Be careful not to arch your back excessively.

Instead of using a band, you can also do the stretch manually (see the illustration on the following page).

2 While on your knees, lean slowly backward, supporting yourself with your hands on the floor. Place your feet far enough apart so they do not interfere with your descent. When you are flexible enough, you can rest your back on the floor, but be careful not to arch your back too much.

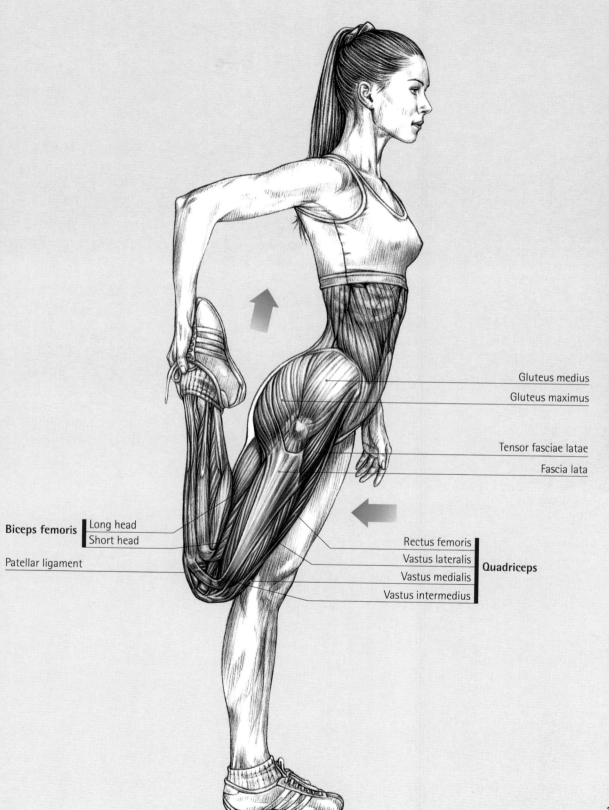

Gluteus medius

Gluteus maximus

Tensor fasciae latae

Fascia lata

Biceps femoris | Long head
Short head

Rectus femoris

Vastus lateralis

Vastus medialis

Vastus intermedius

Quadriceps

Patellar ligament

169

STRENGTHEN YOUR LEGS
Hamstrings

▌Role of the Hamstrings

The hamstrings (the backs of the thighs) are muscles for movement. Except for a small section, they are multijoint muscles. When you walk, run, or jump, you stretch them at one end and contract them at the other end. Their length varies only slightly despite this muscle contraction, which allows them to stay very powerful and very quick during any movement.

The hamstrings are therefore very useful in most sports, since they are the muscles (with the aid of the quadriceps, the glutes, and the calves) that help you move as quickly as possible.

Despite their key role in daily life, the hamstrings are really neglected aesthetically because they cannot be seen from the front.

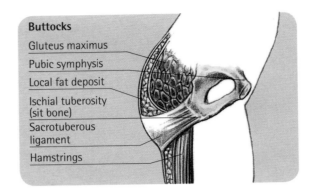

Buttocks
- Gluteus maximus
- Pubic symphysis
- Local fat deposit
- Ischial tuberosity (sit bone)
- Sacrotuberous ligament
- Hamstrings

However, the hamstrings provide a very distinct shaping to the thigh. The upper hamstrings are also located where a large amount of ugly fat normally appears. This occurs especially in women, even though some men have fat here that resembles cellulite. If this is a problem for you, then working the hamstrings, especially in long sets, is an absolute necessity.

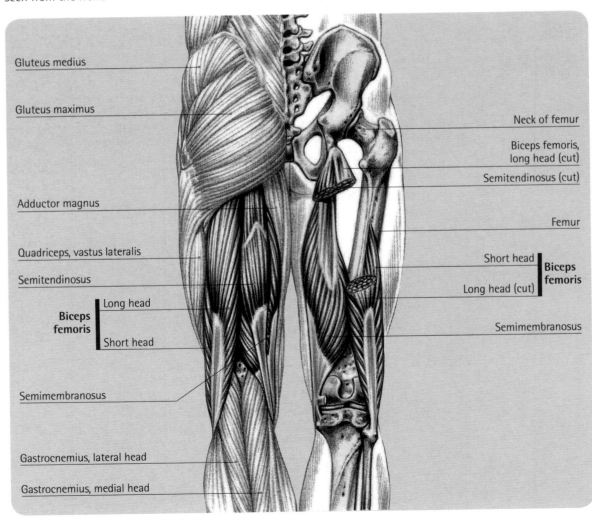

Gluteus medius

Gluteus maximus

Neck of femur

Biceps femoris, long head (cut)

Semitendinosus (cut)

Femur

Adductor magnus

Quadriceps, vastus lateralis

Short head | Biceps femoris
Long head (cut)

Semitendinosus

Biceps femoris
Long head

Short head

Semimembranosus

Semimembranosus

Gastrocnemius, lateral head

Gastrocnemius, medial head

LEGS

170

/// Straight-Legged Deadlift

This isolation exercise works the hamstrings, glutes, and lumbar muscles.
It can be done unilaterally on one leg.

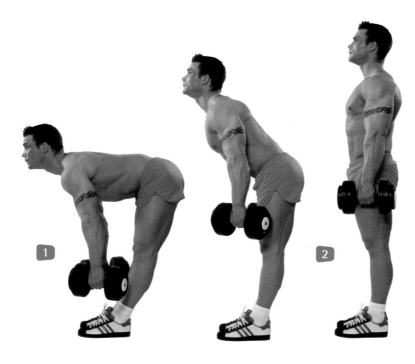

1 With your feet together, bend over and pick up two dumbbells that you have placed on the floor. Keep your back straight and very slightly arched backward. Use a natural hand grip. The ideal is a semipronated grip—a grip somewhere between a neutral grip (thumbs forward) and a pronated grip (thumbs facing each other).

2 Stand up, keeping your legs semistraight. Once you are standing, bend forward while keeping the legs straight to return to your starting position.

! The spine is heavily worked in this exercise. Even though curving your back will give you a larger range of motion, it is still better to keep your spine very straight, slightly arched backward, even if this means you cannot go as low as you would like. You can protect your back by bending the legs just a little instead of keeping them perfectly straight.

Variations

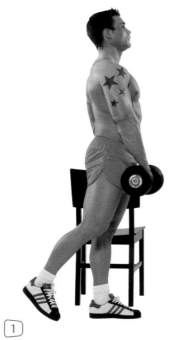

1 You can do this exercise on only one leg, which will keep your spine from having to support too much weight. Hold onto a chair or a wall. Leave your left foot on the floor and extend your right leg out behind you.

2 Lean your torso forward. Ideally, if you are flexible enough, you can lean forward until your torso is parallel with the floor. Then stand up using the strength of your hamstrings and your glutes. Once you have finished a set on the left leg, then move to the right leg.

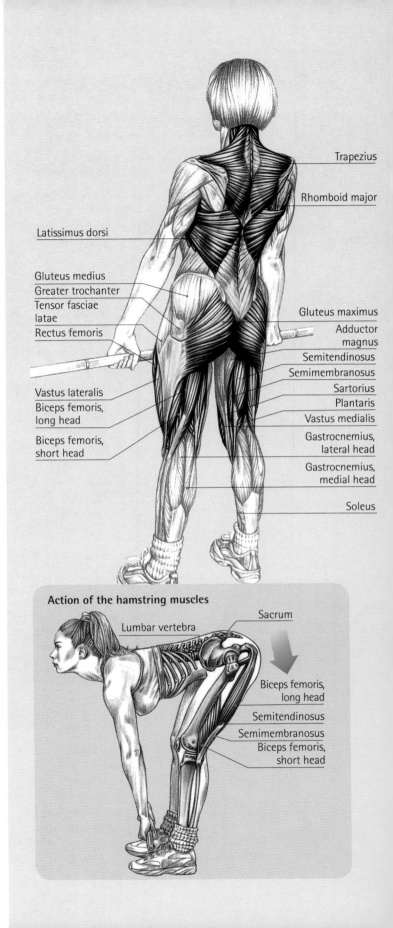

HELPFUL HINTS

When the lumbar muscles get tired, it becomes more and more difficult to maintain the slight natural arch of the back. The spine will start to curve. In this case, reduce the range of motion so that you can always keep your back straight and maintain muscular tension in the hamstrings.

Ideally, you should not bring your torso up until it is perpendicular to the floor. By not coming all the way up, you maintain continuous tension in the hamstrings. Only at failure should you come all the way up and rest for a few seconds so that you can then do a few more repetitions.

NOTES

If at first the straight-legged deadlift seems like an easy exercise for you, remember that it is a much more dangerous exercise than it appears. It is difficult to maintain both balance and good technical execution. If you bend the spine and pull excessively with your back rather than use your hamstrings, you could use more weight or do more repetitions, but this kind of poor technique will reduce the workload on your hamstrings and will make this exercise very dangerous.

ADVANTAGES

This exercise stretches the hamstrings intensely. It puts the hamstrings in a position that is little used in daily life, and that means it might cause serious aches and pains.

Even though it resembles the classic deadlift, the straight-legged version is not a multijoint exercise, so it does not take advantage of the fact that the hamstrings are multijoint muscles.

DISADVANTAGES

LEGS

Trapezius

Rhomboid major

Latissimus dorsi

Gluteus medius
Greater trochanter
Tensor fasciae latae
Rectus femoris

Gluteus maximus

Adductor magnus

Semitendinosus

Semimembranosus

Sartorius

Plantaris

Vastus medialis

Vastus lateralis
Biceps femoris, long head

Biceps femoris, short head

Gastrocnemius, lateral head

Gastrocnemius, medial head

Soleus

Action of the hamstring muscles

Lumbar vertebra

Sacrum

Biceps femoris, long head

Semitendinosus

Semimembranosus

Biceps femoris, short head

/// Seated Leg Curl

This is an isolation exercise for the hamstrings. You can do seated leg curls unilaterally if you need to develop the backs of your thighs.

1 Attach a band to a fixed object on the floor in front of you (for example, a pull-up bar that you have placed at that height). Put the other end of the band around your ankles.

Sit on the tallest chair you have so that your feet are not touching the floor. You can even put a cushion on the chair if you need more height. Hold onto the chair with your hands and keep your legs straight.

Do not lift the legs when you are leaning forward. This could stretch your hamstring muscles too much.

2 Use your hamstring muscles to bring your feet as far under the chair as possible. Hold this contracted position for two to three seconds before straightening your legs.

(Variations)

You can work one leg at a time. You can also vary the width of your legs. In the basic position, you keep your legs squeezed together, but you can separate them if you want to. The only issue with this is that you might end up hitting your feet on the chair.

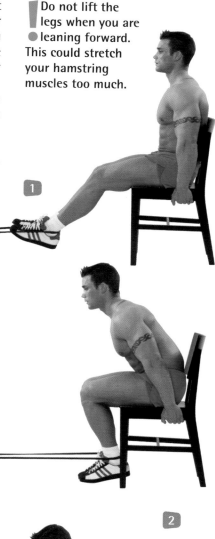

HELPFUL HINTS

The secret of this exercise is in the movement of the torso. When your legs are straight, your back is straight. The farther you bring your legs under the chair, the more you lean forward. While the legs are bending to 90 degrees, the torso is bending to 45 degrees. The reverse happens when you extend your legs. You will notice that you are much stronger this way and that you feel the back of the thighs working more. In fact, moving the torso stretches the hamstrings near the glutes and shortens them near the knees. This is the optimal way for the hamstrings to work.

NOTES

If you typically have trouble feeling work in your hamstrings, then use seated leg curls as a preexhaustion exercise before straight-legged deadlifts. In this way you will be able to feel the effects of the deadlifts. In addition, since you have already tired out the hamstrings, you can use less weight during the deadlifts, which is better for your spine.

ADVANTAGES

Even though this is technically an isolation exercise, the seated leg curl becomes a multijoint exercise if you really move your torso well. This optimizes the length-tension relationship of the multijoint muscle in the back of the thigh.

- - - - - - - - - - - -

If you do not move your torso, you will arch your back when you contract your hamstrings. This arch will put your spine in an awkward position for no reason at all. The tension created in the back during this exercise demonstrates that there is no physiological reason to stay firmly seated on a chair during the entire exercise. Moreover, you will have great difficulty in bringing your feet under your body if you keep your torso too straight.

DISADVANTAGES

/// Lying Leg Curl

This is an isolation exercise for the hamstrings. It can be done unilaterally, but only with a band.

! Arching your back will make you stronger, but it will compress the discs in your lumbar spine.

You must carefully control your dumbbell because you could be seriously injured if it slips.

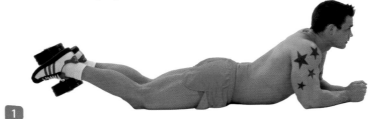

1

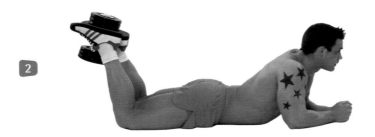

2

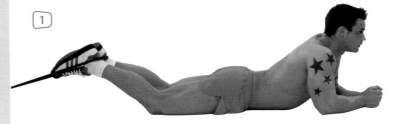

1

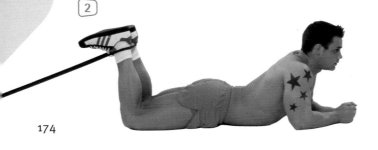

2

1 While standing, grip a dumbbell between your feet. Then lie face-down on the floor or a bed (with your knees on the edge so that your dumbbell does not hit the floor when you straighten your legs).

2 Using your hamstrings, bring the dumbbell up to your buttocks. At some point near the top of the movement, you will feel that there is no more resistance on the muscle. This loss of tension means it is time to stop the movement upward and reverse the direction so that you maintain continuous tension on the muscle.

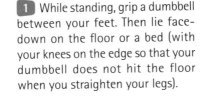

HELPFUL HINTS
Begin slowly with a light weight so that you get used to gripping the dumbbell securely. Perform this exercise in a slow and controlled manner, not explosively.

(Variations)

1 **2** Instead of using a dumbbell, you can use a band attached to the floor to create resistance. There are two benefits to this:

1. It is easier to hold a band with your ankles than it is to hold a dumbbell.
2. Tension remains continuous for the whole exercise, especially at the end.

Ideally, you could combine a dumbbell and a band, but setting that up might be difficult unless you are working out with a partner.

LEGS

174

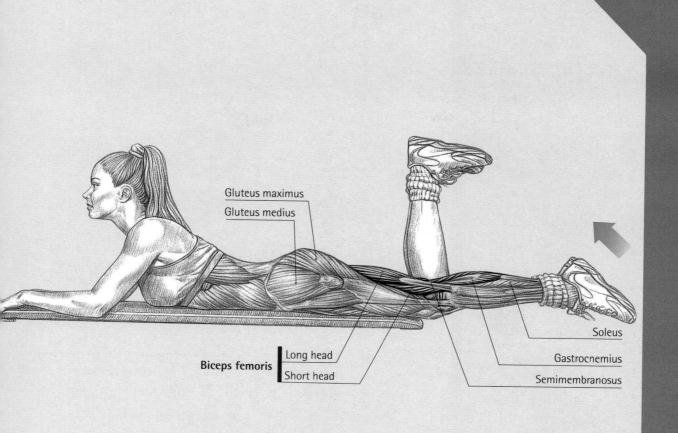

Gluteus maximus

Gluteus medius

Soleus

Gastrocnemius

Semimembranosus

Biceps femoris | Long head

Short head

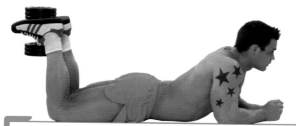

NOTES

The position of your toes plays an important role in contracting the hamstrings. If you flex your toes toward your knees, you will be stronger because the power of your calves will combine with that of your hamstrings. But this gain in strength means that you lose the good isolation work on the hamstrings.

However, if you keep your toes pointed up as much as possible, you will have less strength, but you will isolate the hamstrings more.

One strategy is to begin the exercise with your toes pointed up as much as possible. At failure, flex your feet to bring the toes toward the knees. This change will give you more strength by recruiting the calf muscles. You can then do a few more repetitions.

ADVANTAGES

This exercise really isolates the back of the thigh, and it helps you immediately feel this muscle.

- - - - - - - - - - - - - - - - - - -

Leg curls do not take advantage of the fact that the hamstrings are multijoint muscles. The non-physiological aspect of this exercise explains the natural tendency to arch the back and lift the glutes during the contraction. This multijoint nature of the hamstrings shows through in this artificial exercise. This anatomical conflict puts the back in an unstable position.

DISADVANTAGES

/// Stretching the Hamstrings

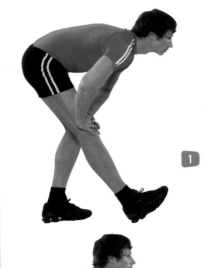

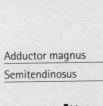

Gluteus maximus

Adductor magnus
Semitendinosus

Quadriceps | Vastus lateralis
| Rectus femoris

Biceps femoris | Long head
| Short head

Quadriceps,
vastus intermedius
Semimembranosus

Triceps surae | Gastrocnemius, medial head
| Gastrocnemius, lateral head
| Soleus

LEGS

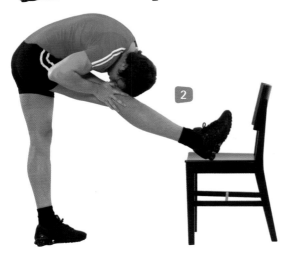

1 Place one heel on the floor, a chair, or a table (the higher your foot, the greater the stretch). Straighten the leg and put your hands on the stretched thigh, a little above the knee.

2 Slowly bend forward. When your hamstring is really stretched, you can bend your standing leg a little to get an even better stretch.

Calves

Role of the Calves

In athletic endeavors, the calves play the biggest role in running or jumping. They are therefore very important in most sports.

Aesthetically, they provide the finishing touch to the shape of the legs. They are sometimes difficult to develop and are often neglected.

The calves consist of two muscles:
1. The **gastrocnemius** provides most of the muscle mass of the calf.
2. The **soleus** is covered by the gastrocnemius. It has much less mass than the gastrocnemius.

Other than size, there is a great difference between the gastrocnemius and the soleus. Only the gastrocnemius is a multijoint muscle. This particularity will have serious repercussions for every calf exercise.

Because it is a single-joint muscle, the soleus participates in all calf exercises whether or not the leg is bent. However, the more you bend your leg, the less the gastrocnemius will be able to assist with that movement. This is why exercises in which the leg is bent at 90 degrees will isolate the soleus and neglect the gastrocnemius.

To really work the gastrocnemius, the leg must be nearly straight. Ideally, the knee is slightly bent and the torso is leaning forward, a position used in donkey calf raises.

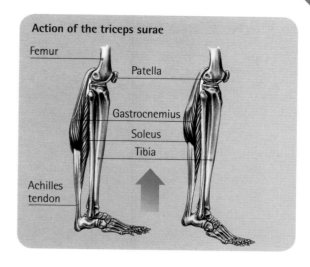

Action of the triceps surae

Femur · Patella · Gastrocnemius · Soleus · Tibia · Achilles tendon

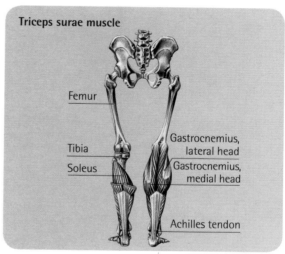

Triceps surae muscle

Femur · Tibia · Soleus · Gastrocnemius, lateral head · Gastrocnemius, medial head · Achilles tendon

! It is often recommended that you straighten your legs completely in order to work the gastrocnemius muscles. This is a mistake. The gastrocnemius muscle is stronger when the knee is slightly bent because, in that position, the length–tension relationship provides more strength than when the leg is totally straight. Moreover, it is hard to see why nature would have required us to straighten our legs perfectly to get the most strength out of our gastrocnemius muscles.

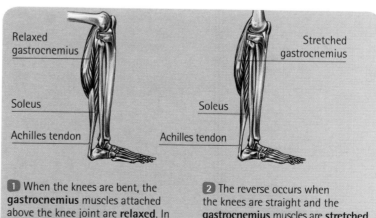

Relaxed gastrocnemius · Soleus · Achilles tendon — Stretched gastrocnemius · Soleus · Achilles tendon

1 When the knees are bent, the **gastrocnemius** muscles attached above the knee joint are **relaxed**. In this position, they participate weakly in extending the feet; most of the work is done by the **soleus** muscles.

2 The reverse occurs when the knees are straight and the **gastrocnemius** muscles are **stretched**. In this position, they actively participate in extending the feet and they complement the work of the soleus muscles.

/// Standing Calf Raise

This isolation exercise targets the whole calf and the gastrocnemius muscle in particular.
It can be done unilaterally. It works the calf using the weight of the whole body. Working only one calf at a time provides a better stretch and better contraction of the muscle, which increases the range of motion.

LEGS

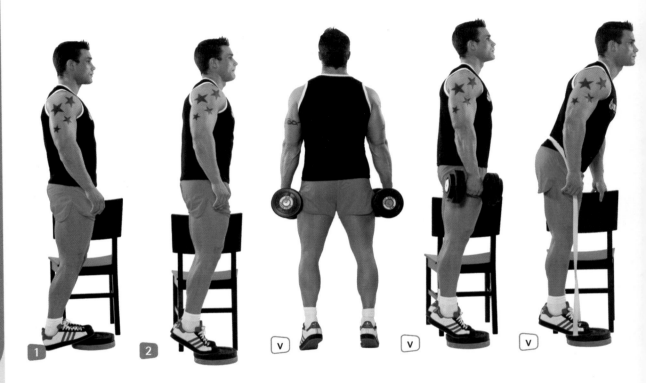

1 Put the balls of your feet (or one foot) on a weight plate or board. Stretch the calves to their maximum before rising up as high as you can onto the balls of your feet.

2 Hold the contracted position for one second before lowering your heels to the floor. You may hold onto a chair or the wall to help maintain your balance.

Variations

v You can turn your feet out or in, but it is better to keep them straight in line with your legs to avoid unnecessary twisting of your knees, especially if you are using weights to increase the muscle work. In any case, the orientation of your feet will not change the basic shape of your calves.

However, turning the feet out or in reduces the calves' strength and also the effectiveness of the exercise. The calves will be strongest when your feet are pointing straight ahead. If you absolutely must do a variation, then alter the width of the feet (narrow or wide) rather than their orientation.

You can use a band or one or two dumbbells plus a band to increase the resistance.

178

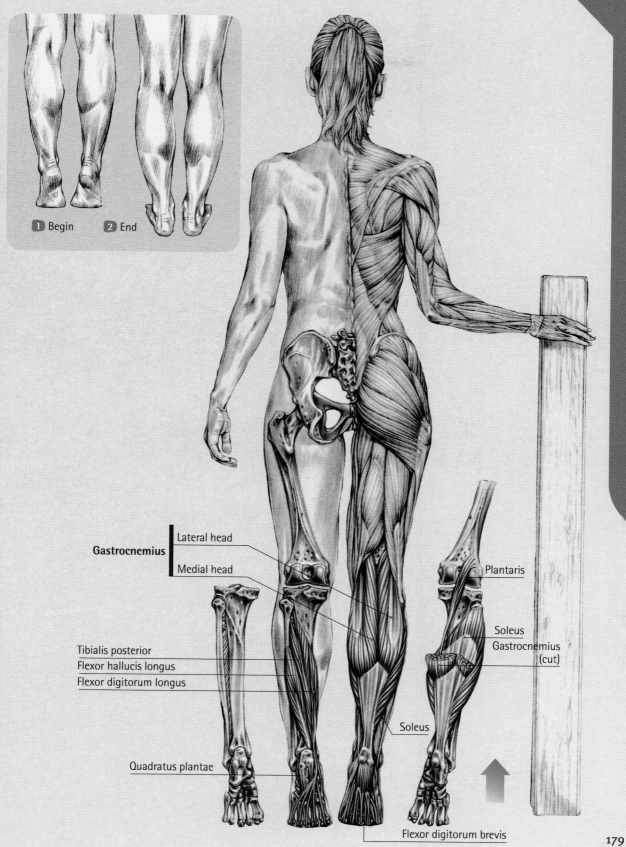

1 Begin 2 End

Gastrocnemius — Lateral head

Medial head

Plantaris

Soleus

Gastrocnemius (cut)

Tibialis posterior

Flexor hallucis longus

Flexor digitorum longus

Soleus

Quadratus plantae

Flexor digitorum brevis

179

> Adding weight will create pressure on the spine. Work only one calf at a time so that you do not need to add much resistance.

ADVANTAGES

This exercise is great for focused work on the calf.

- - - - - - - - - - - - - - - - - - -

This exercise does not stretch the calf as well as donkey calf raises (see page 181). It also does not put the calf into an optimal position to benefit from the length-tension relationship.

DISADVANTAGES

HELPFUL HINTS

You must absolutely avoid moving the buttocks from front to back by arching your lower back. These tiny movements are often the result of keeping the legs too straight, especially in the stretched position.

NOTES

People often describe standing calf raises as a multijoint exercise, but that is incorrect since the exercise only works the ankle joint.

LEGS

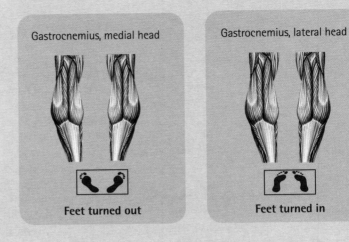

Gastrocnemius, medial head

Feet turned out

Gastrocnemius, lateral head

Feet turned in

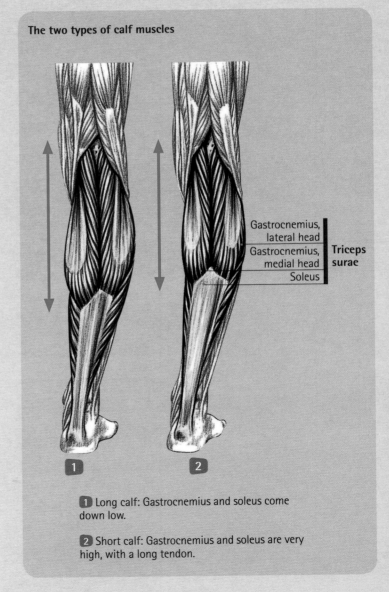

The two types of calf muscles

Gastrocnemius, lateral head
Gastrocnemius, medial head
Soleus
Triceps surae

1 Long calf: Gastrocnemius and soleus come down low.

2 Short calf: Gastrocnemius and soleus are very high, with a long tendon.

/// Donkey Calf Raise

This isolation exercise works the whole calf, particularly the gastrocnemius muscle. It can be done unilaterally, which will work the calf using the weight of your whole body. Also, working only one calf at a time means you can stretch and contract the muscle better.

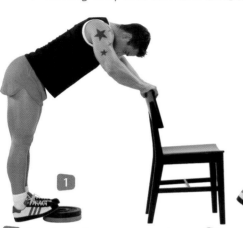

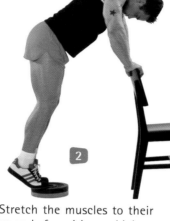

1 Put the balls of your feet (or one foot) on a weight plate, board, or phone book. Lean forward so that your torso forms a 90- to 110-degree angle with the floor. Place your hands on the back of a chair to support your torso.

! If you have a partner or an elastic band to provide resistance, be sure that the weight is placed on your hips as much as possible (rather than on your spine) so that you do not have unnecessary pressure on your back.

2 Stretch the muscles to their maximum before rising as high as possible onto the balls of your feet. Hold the contracted position for one second before lowering your heels to the floor.

HELPFUL HINTS
Do not keep your legs too straight, especially when you are standing up on the balls of your feet.

NOTES
People often describe this as a multijoint exercise, but that is not correct since the exercise involves only the ankle joint.

Variations

1 If you have a partner, he can sit on the edge of your lower back. Incidentally, this is how the exercise got its name.

2 If you do not have a partner, you can use a dumbbell or a band. Hold the band under the front of your feet and put the other end around your hips.

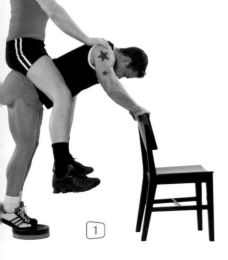

1

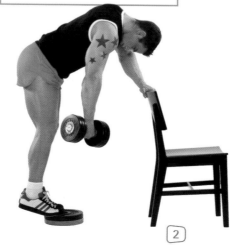

2

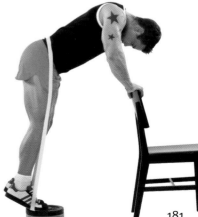

181

/// Sit Squat

This isolation exercise primarily works the soleus muscle and, to a lesser degree, the gastrocnemius muscle. It is not a good idea to do this exercise unilaterally.

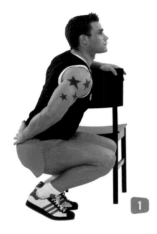

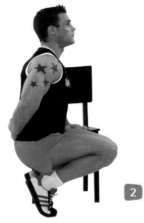

! This exercise has little to no risk associated with it.

1 Crouch with the balls of your feet on a phone book, a board, a weight plate, or the floor. Hold on tightly to a chair with one or both hands. Stretch your calves to their maximum.

2 Lift up onto the balls of your feet as high as you can. Hold the contracted position for one second before lowering your heels to the floor.

Variations

Vary the width of your feet rather than their orientation to increase the diversity of this exercise.

HELPFUL HINTS

The calves are meant to be resisting muscles rather than power muscles. For this reason it is better to work them in long sets (20 to 25 repetitions per set).

NOTES

A good superset is to begin with sit squats, and at failure, stand up and do standing calf raises followed by donkey calf raises.

ADVANTAGES

There is no tension in the lumbar region. Unlike other calf exercises, you can rise very high onto the balls of your feet, and this will help you achieve an intense muscular contraction. Take full advantage of this fact.

- - - - - - - - - - - - - - - - - -

It is not very easy to increase resistance during this exercise, but you can try putting a weight plate on your thighs. It is easier to increase the range of motion (in both the stretching and contracting phases) than it is to add weight.

DISADVANTAGES

LEGS

/// Seated Calf Raise

This is an isolation exercise especially for the soleus. It can be done unilaterally.

! To avoid injuring your knees, do not place resistance (dumbbells or weight plates) directly on them. Move the weight up about two inches on the thigh. Do not move the weight any higher, since that would make the exercise too easy.

HELPFUL HINTS

To go as high as possible onto the balls of your feet, you need to be sure to move all the resistance from your big toes to your small toes at the end of the movement.

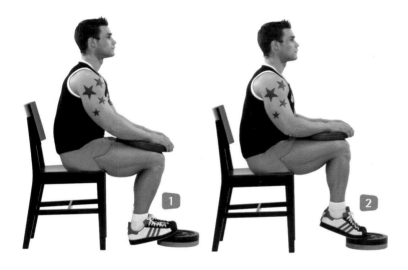

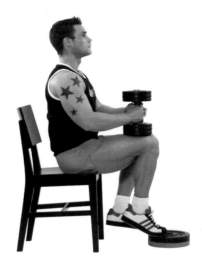

1 Sit on a chair or a bed and put the balls of your feet on a weight plate, board, or phone book. Weight, such as a weight plate or one or two dumbbells placed on your lower thighs, will provide resistance.

2 Rise up as high as possible onto the balls of your feet. Hold the contracted position for one second before lowering your heels to the floor.

You can also exercise just one calf at a time.

Variations

If your goal is to reproduce the kind of muscle work that occurs when you are running, you can work each calf alternately: When one calf is contracted, the other is stretched. To do this, put a dumbbell on each of your thighs so that the calves can work independently.

COMMENTS

This exercise is especially worthwhile in sports that require jumping and running.

ADVANTAGES

This exercise is relatively easy because it does not work large muscle masses. It does not create any tension in the lumbar region.

- - - - - - - - - - - - - - - -

This is a very popular exercise, but it does not work the calves much since the soleus muscles are the only ones working. Because the legs are bent, the gastrocnemius muscles have a hard time assisting with the exercise.

DISADVANTAGES

183

/// Plyometric Exercises for the Calves

The primary plyometric exercise for the calves is jumping on the balls of your feet.

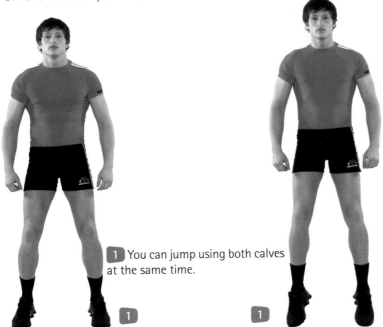

1 You can jump using both calves at the same time.

1

1

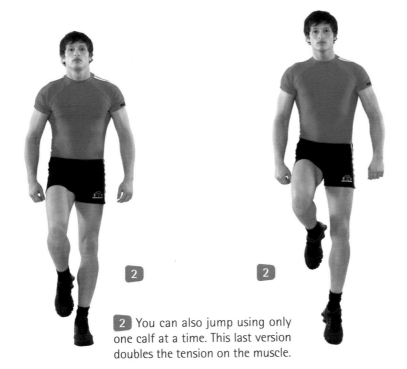

2

2

2 You can also jump using only one calf at a time. This last version doubles the tension on the muscle.

/// Stretching the Calves

You can do calf stretches on a single leg or on both legs at the same time. The range of the stretch is much greater when you stretch one leg at a time because

> you are always more flexible during unilateral stretches, and
> your body weight forces the stretch much more when the weight is applied to one leg rather than distributed on both legs.

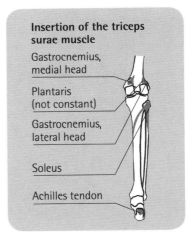

Insertion of the triceps surae muscle

Gastrocnemius, medial head

Plantaris (not constant)

Gastrocnemius, lateral head

Soleus

Achilles tendon

There are many angles from which you can stretch your calf muscles. A very straight leg will primarily stretch the gastrocnemius muscle. A bent leg will stretch the soleus muscle. It is important for athletes to stretch their calves thoroughly from all angles (standing, lunging, and twisting) because each exercise stretches distinctly different parts of the calf. These exercises are complementary and in no way redundant.

1 Standing. Put the balls of your feet (or one foot) on a weight plate, board, or phone book. The higher the object, the greater the stretch you will feel. Hold the position for 12 seconds.

❗ Athletes need to keep the feet very flexible in order to avoid hurting the ankles. You should always begin any workout for your particular sport with calf stretches.

It is also essential to keep your ankles flexible so that you will be able to keep your back as straight as possible during thigh exercises such as the squat. The calves are attached to the femurs, so it is important to stretch the calves before working the quadriceps or the hamstrings in order to properly warm up the knee joints.

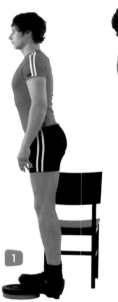

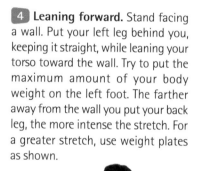

3 Sitting with a band.

4 Leaning forward. Stand facing a wall. Put your left leg behind you, keeping it straight, while leaning your torso toward the wall. Try to put the maximum amount of your body weight on the left foot. The farther away from the wall you put your back leg, the more intense the stretch. For a greater stretch, use weight plates as shown.

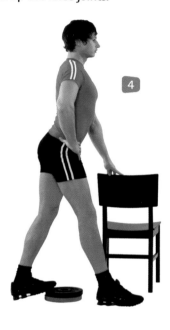

2 Lunging. Do a forward lunge while the ball of the front foot is on a weight, board, or phone book. The farther forward you place your knee, the more intense the stretch. Slowly bring most of your body weight over the foot that you are stretching.

5 Twisting the ankle to the side. This is a stretch for the muscles on the outside of the calves. These are the same muscles that you strain if you twist your ankle. Since the slightest excessive stretch of these muscles will prevent you from playing your sport, it is important to work on flexibility to prevent injuries.

Stand with your feet close together and put your weight on your left foot. Roll your right foot as far over to the side as possible. Slowly move your weight over to the right foot. You should do this stretch progressively and slowly so that you do not tear a muscle or a tendon. Once you have stretched the right foot, repeat the stretch on the left foot.

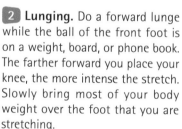

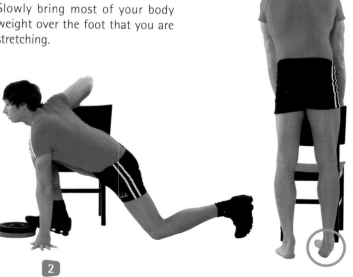

FIRM UP YOUR GLUTES

▌Role of the Glutes

The glutes support the hamstrings when you need to increase your speed. When you walk slowly, they work very little, but as soon as you accelerate, they are recruited. When you run, they put forth their maximum effort. The glutes are therefore very important in sports that require rapid movement or jumping.

Aesthetically, the glutes have a unique purpose. Large arms may be impressive, but a shapely buttocks is attractive to the opposite sex. Women are often considered the only ones to be concerned with the shape of their buttocks, primarily for the shape and secondarily for the firmness. Today, more and more men are realizing the aesthetic importance of their buttocks. They are also searching for ways to firm up their glutes.

Training the glutes for a sport primarily means strengthening the muscles and increasing their explosiveness. Aesthetically, you should not only try to round them but also improve their definition and contour, somewhat similar to what people try to achieve with their abdominal muscles.

NOTE

Squats, lunges, and deadlifts are excellent exercises for the glutes. We will not describe them here since we have already done so in other parts of the book. To better recruit the glutes, though, squeeze your buttocks together tightly throughout the exercises. At first you might have trouble doing this, but after several workouts, you will be able to do it automatically if you are concentrating. You should also lean forward slightly so that the glutes are more involved in the exercises. However, you must pay attention to your back. When you lean forward, you also increase the pressure on your spine.

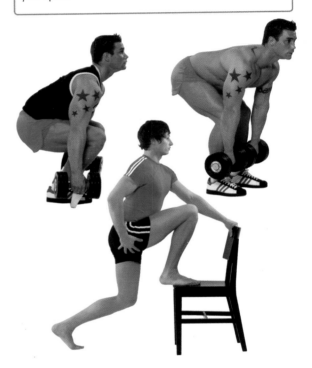

CAN SPORTS MELT AWAY FAT?

Is it possible to lose your belly fat or reduce cellulite by specifically working the abdominal muscles or the glutes? For a long time, medical studies had trouble proving that fat could be eliminated in trouble spots by stimulating the underlying muscles. However, there are two major arguments in favor of spot reduction of fat through weight training exercises done in long sets:

1 Modern studies show that exercise accelerates the loss of fat covering the muscles that are working.

2 Local muscle work increases blood flow to fat deposits. This accelerates the burning of fat and prevents its growth.

To increase the effectiveness of localized weight training, you must combine it with a proper diet. It is also recommended that you do firming exercises, preferably in the morning on an empty stomach and in the evening before going to bed. In the morning and at bedtime, do two to four sets of 20 to 50 repetitions of one of the exercises that we will describe.

If you are not concerned with losing body fat, know that this strategy of targeting muscles can be used as a preventive measure against accumulation of fat deposits. In fact, fat typically accumulates over muscles that are not often used in daily life. The glutes and the abdominal muscles are rarely recruited in daily activities, which results in the typical fat deposits. By taking five minutes in the morning and the evening to work these muscles, you can firm them up and prevent fat from forming.

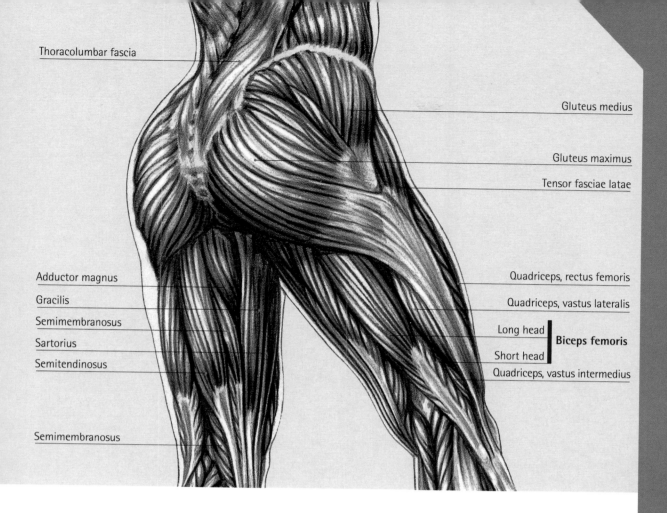

Thoracolumbar fascia

Gluteus medius

Gluteus maximus

Tensor fasciae latae

Adductor magnus

Gracilis

Semimembranosus

Sartorius

Semitendinosus

Semimembranosus

Quadriceps, rectus femoris

Quadriceps, vastus lateralis

Long head
Short head **Biceps femoris**

Quadriceps, vastus intermedius

HOW DOES CELLULITE DEVELOP?

Most women complain of having cellulite. This condition is rarer in men. Five major steps lead to the formation of cellulite:

1 Beginning in adolescence, the production of female hormones (estrogen and progesterone) intensifies. These hormones develop and harden the network of connective tissue that encloses the fat cells, particularly in the lower body.

2 When fat tissue begins to grow, it pushes on the hard connective tissue, which interrupts the local microcirculation of blood.

3 This causes a lack of oxygen, excessive pro-duction of free radicals, and local inflammation.

4 This environment favors the accumulation of fat and the retention of water.

5 The inflammation destroys collagen fibers in the skin. This breakdown makes fat deposits more visible. You can now see the cottage-cheese look of cellulite. It only gets worse with age because aging reduces the density and flexibility of the skin. Using tobacco or birth control pills, which are harmful to collagen, accentuates this phenomenon.

/// Hip Extension

This is an isolation exercise for the glutes, lumbar muscles, and hamstrings. It must be done unilaterally.

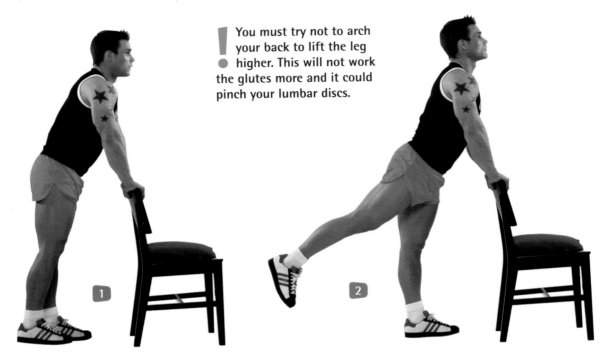

! You must try not to arch your back to lift the leg higher. This will not work the glutes more and it could pinch your lumbar discs.

1 Stand about 6 inches (15 cm) away from a wall or the back of a chair. Put one hand on the wall or the chair to remain very stable. Lean forward.

2 Using your glutes, lift your back leg (which should remain very straight) up as far as possible. Hold the contracted position for one second while squeezing your buttocks together as tightly as possible. Return to the starting position with both legs together. Once you have finished a set on one leg, move immediately to the other leg.

HELPFUL HINTS
To really work the gluteus maximus, do not pivot your torso toward the outside. The exercise will certainly be easier, but its ability to shape the buttocks will be compromised. However, it is normal for the leg to move slightly toward the outside when you stretch it behind you.

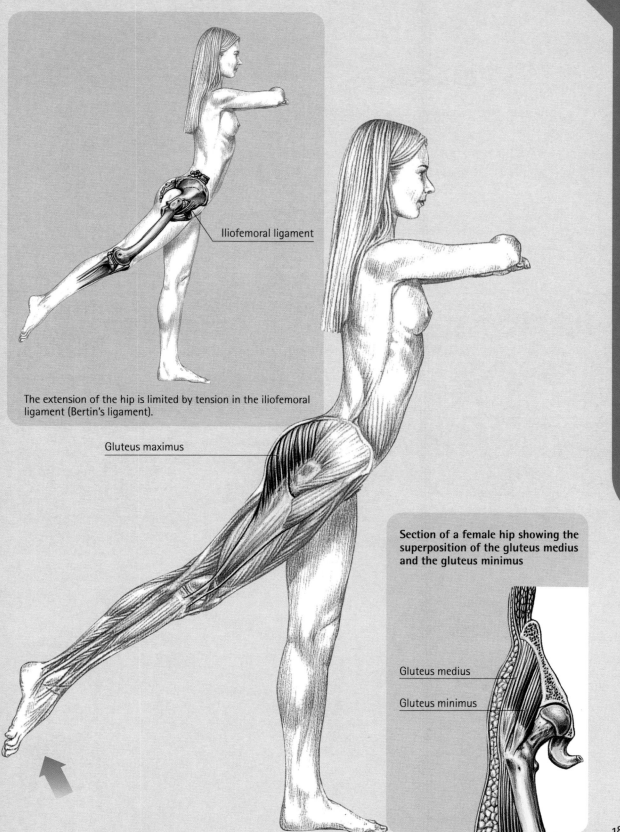

Iliofemoral ligament

The extension of the hip is limited by tension in the iliofemoral ligament (Bertin's ligament).

Gluteus maximus

Section of a female hip showing the superposition of the gluteus medius and the gluteus minimus

Gluteus medius

Gluteus minimus

189

Variations

You can increase the difficulty of this exercise by doing it on all fours on the floor or on a bed. On a bed, you can increase the range of motion by moving to the edge of the mattress and allowing your working leg to descend as low as possible.

ADVANTAGES

This exercise isolates the glutes very well. You will feel the muscle working right away.

- - - - - - - - - - - - - - - - -

Compared to multijoint exercises like the squat, you lose a lot of time because you can work only one thigh at a time.

DISADVANTAGES

1 If you do the exercise on the floor, you should bend your leg to 90 degrees so that you can bring it under your torso to increase the range of motion.

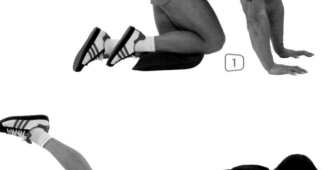

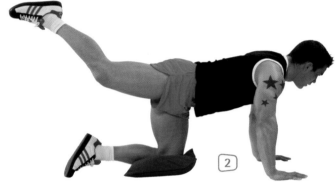

2 Straighten the leg out again as soon as it is no longer underneath you.

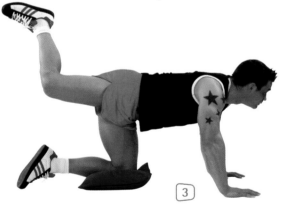

3 At failure, you can keep the leg bent to 90 degrees throughout the exercise. This will make the exercise easier and allow you to do a few more repetitions.

TIP
To better feel your muscle working, rest your right hand on the right glutes when they are contracting. Touching the muscles improves the brain–muscle connection, which increases muscle sensation and makes the work that much more productive.

NOTES
When standing, you can add resistance by putting a band around your ankles.

4 On all fours, put one end of the band around the ankle of your resting leg and the other end around your working thigh, an inch or so above your knee.

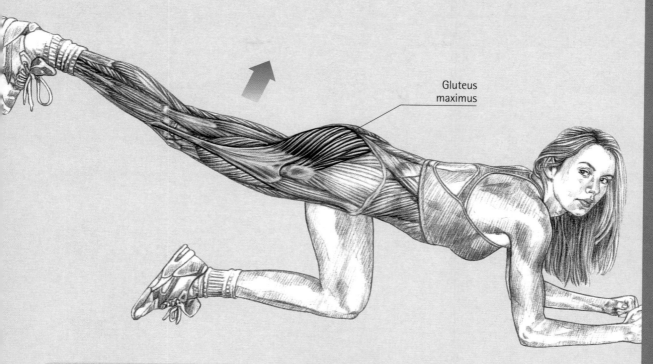

Gluteus maximus

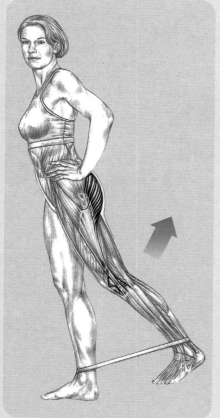

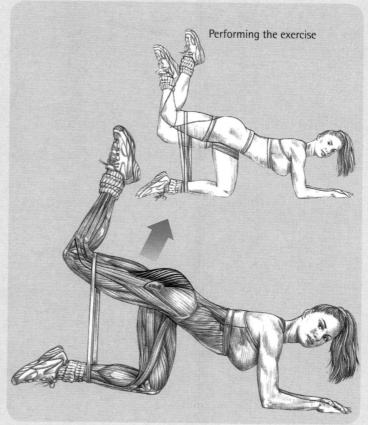

Performing the exercise

/// Lateral Leg Raise (Abduction)

This is an isolation exercise for the gluteus medius and gluteus minimus.
It must be done unilaterally.

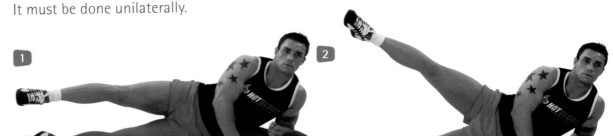

1 Lying on the floor or on a bed on your left side, either support your head with your left hand or rest your left elbow on the floor. The other arm should be bent in front of your abdomen, with your hand flat on the floor for the most stability.

2 Keep your right leg straight and lift it up as high as possible using the strength of your glutes. Hold the contracted position for one second while contracting the right glutes as much as possible. Return to the starting position with both legs practically touching (but not all the way). Once you have finished the exercise on the right leg, move immediately to the left leg.

Variations

1 **2** You can also do this exercise while standing, but there is less resistance this way.

! Do not lift your leg too high, because past a certain height, the glutes stop working and the oblique muscles (the lateral part of the abdominal muscles) take over. Moreover, lifting your leg very high twists the spine and could cause pinching in the lumbar discs.

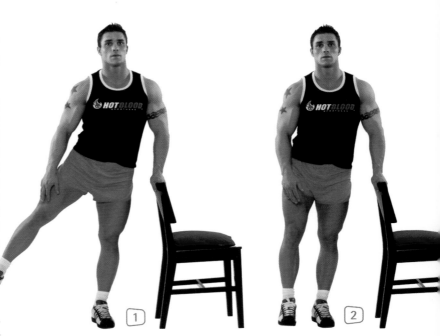

COMMENTS
To increase resistance, you can attach a band to both of your ankles.

A possible combination is to begin the exercise lying down with a band, and at failure, remove the band. When you reach failure again, do a few standing repetitions.

HELPFUL HINTS
You should squeeze the working glutes tightly throughout the entire exercise. To maintain continuous tension in the muscles, do not bring your working leg all the way down against the resting leg.

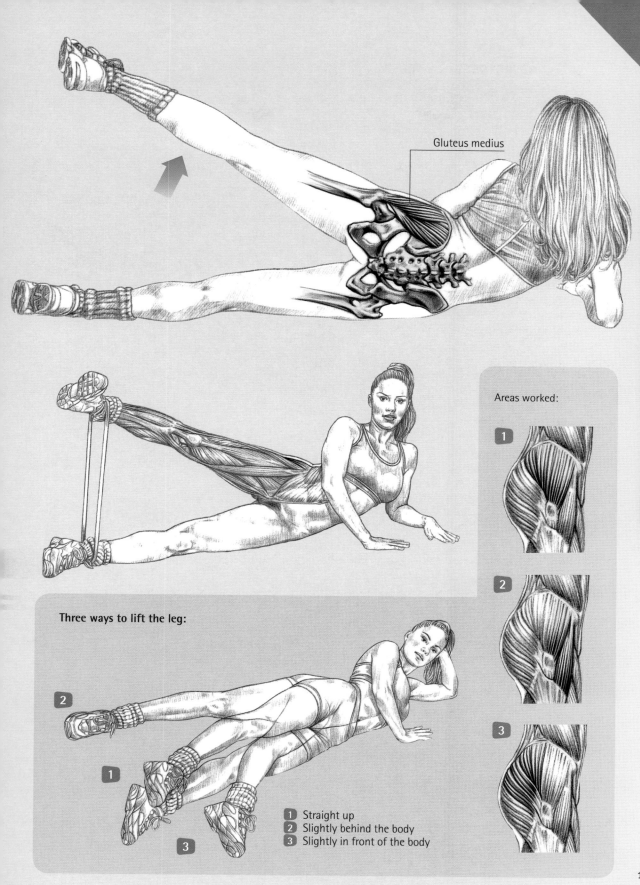

Gluteus medius

Areas worked:

1

2

3

Three ways to lift the leg:

2

1

3

1 Straight up
2 Slightly behind the body
3 Slightly in front of the body

To overcome the "flat butt" phenomenon, this localized work will
create a curve on the upper part of
the buttocks.

This exercise takes a lot of time
and works only a small part of the
glutes.

NOTES

To better feel your muscles working,
place your free hand on the upper part
of the working glutes.

Variations

1 2 You can increase the difficulty of this exercise by doing it
on all fours. To do this, instead of
keeping the leg straight, you will
keep it bent to 90 degrees. It is more
difficult to feel the muscle working
during this version. Even though it
is popular, this version is not better
than the simpler, classic version.

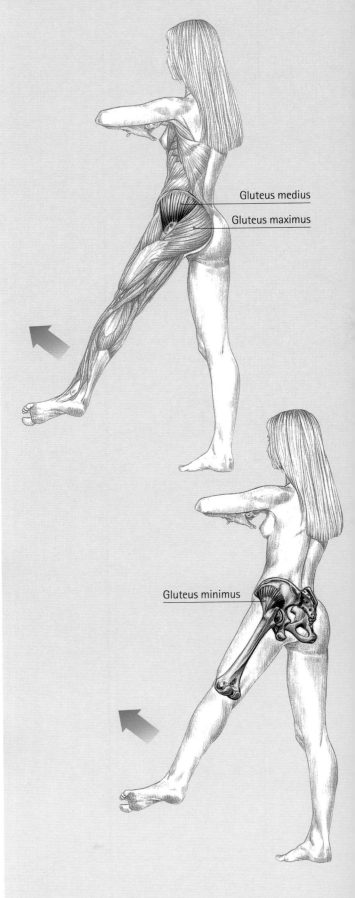

Gluteus medius

Gluteus maximus

Gluteus minimus

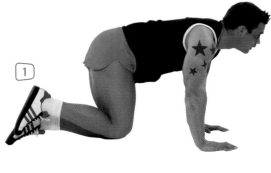

1

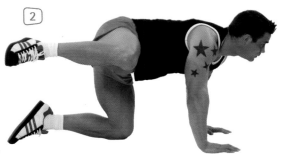

2

GLUTES

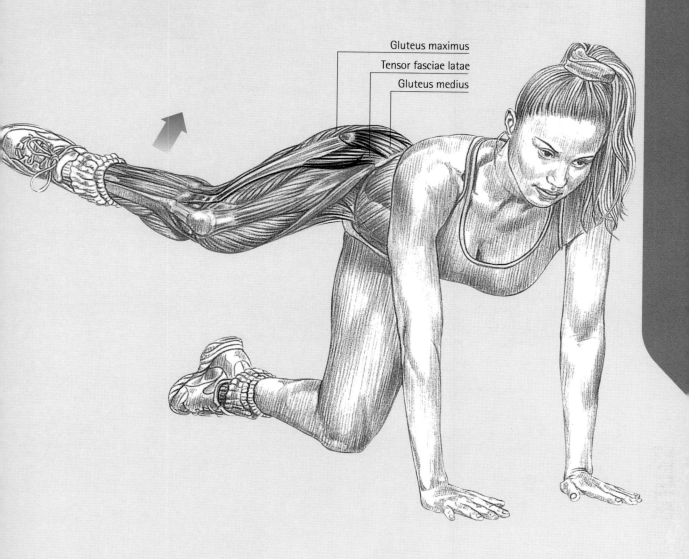

Gluteus maximus

Tensor fasciae latae

Gluteus medius

195

/// Bridge

This is an isolation exercise for the glutes, lumbar muscles, and hamstrings.
This exercise can be done unilaterally.

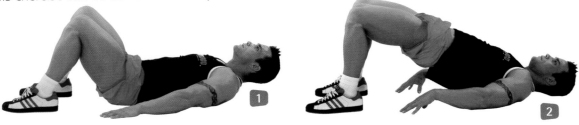

HELPFUL HINTS
You can move your feet closer to or farther away from your buttocks, and you can also vary their width to change the muscles worked during the exercise. With the feet close to the buttocks, it is generally easier to feel the contraction of the glutes.

TIP
Put your hands on the sides of your glutes so that you can better feel them working.

1 Lie on your back on the floor or on a bed with your arms alongside your body and your feet about shoulder-width apart. Bend your knees to 90 degrees and place your feet close to your buttocks.

! ● Do not arch your back to raise your torso higher. You could pinch your lumbar and cervical discs if you do. Unlike the woman you see modeling this exercise in the illustrations on page 197, you should not turn your head to the side. Rather, you should look at the ceiling so that you do not damage your cervical spine.

2 Using your glutes, lift your torso and legs as high as possible so that they form a triangle with the floor. Your shoulders stay on the floor to provide leverage. Hold this potion for one second while squeezing your buttocks as tightly as possible. Return to the starting position.

Repeat the exercise without resting your torso on the floor. When you reach failure, you can pause briefly on the floor to give your muscles a break, and then do a few more repetitions.

NOTES
Squats and bridges are good complementary exercises. A preexhaustion superset is a set of bridges followed by a set of squats.

A postexhaustion superset (squats followed by bridges) helps you really tire out the thighs and increase the number of repetitions during the set.

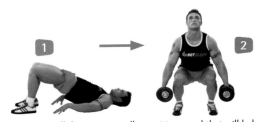

In this way you will do more overall repetitions, and that will help firm up your buttocks. Your back will also be spared because you will not have to use as heavy a weight during squats.

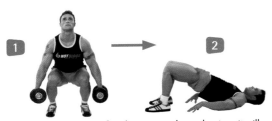

This is a better superset for shaping your buttocks since it will not affect the heavy work done during squats.

GLUTES

196

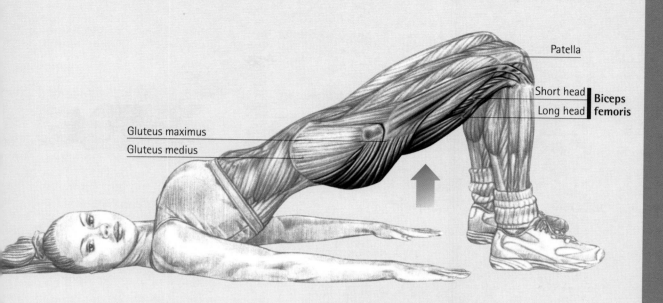

Patella

Short head | **Biceps**
Long head | **femoris**

Gluteus maximus
Gluteus medius

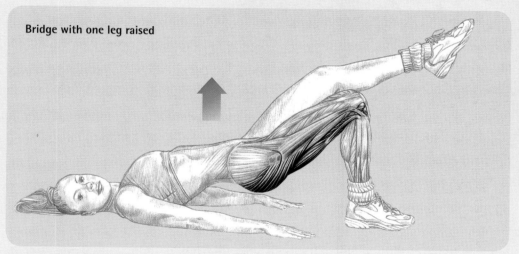

Bridge with one leg raised

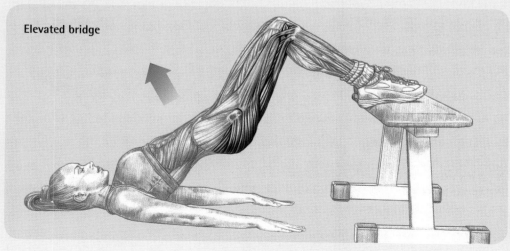

Elevated bridge

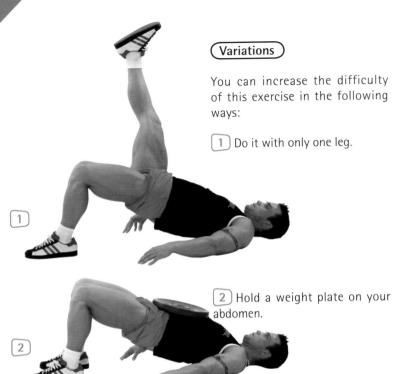

Variations

You can increase the difficulty of this exercise in the following ways:

1 Do it with only one leg.

2 Hold a weight plate on your abdomen.

3 Put your feet on a chair or on the edge of a bed rather than on the floor. In this way, the range of motion is increased because of a better stretch in the glutes.

You can combine two or all three of the variations for maximum effectiveness.

You can also begin the exercise on a chair with a weight (hold the weight with your hands so it does not slip). At failure, put the weight down. When you reach failure again, continue the exercise with your feet on the floor.

ADVANTAGES

Both right and left glutes work simultaneously, so you do not lose any time as you do with unilateral exercises.

- - - - - - - - - - - - - - - -

People with spine problems must be careful with this exercise since it does require a certain amount of flexibility in the spine.

DISADVANTAGES

/// Stretching the Glutes

Lunges are an excellent way to stretch the glutes.

1 Instead of putting your foot on the floor in front of you, put it on a chair to increase the range of the stretch. For best use of this range of motion, bend your back leg so you can drop your buttocks lower than your elevated foot.

In general, exercises that stretch the hamstrings also increase flexibility in the glutes.

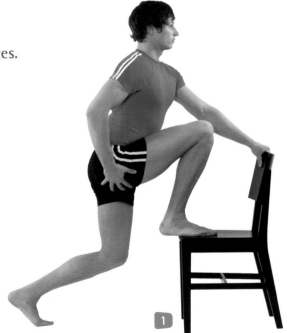

GLUTES

198

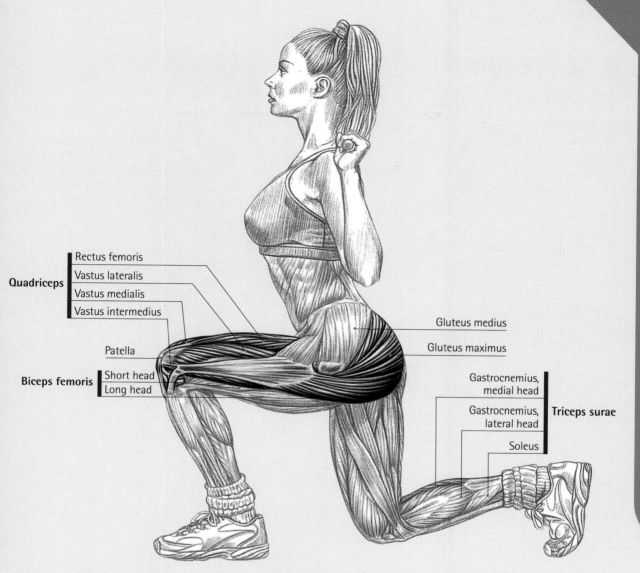

Quadriceps
- Rectus femoris
- Vastus lateralis
- Vastus medialis
- Vastus intermedius

Patella

Biceps femoris
- Short head
- Long head

Gluteus medius

Gluteus maximus

Gastrocnemius, medial head

Gastrocnemius, lateral head

Soleus

Triceps surae

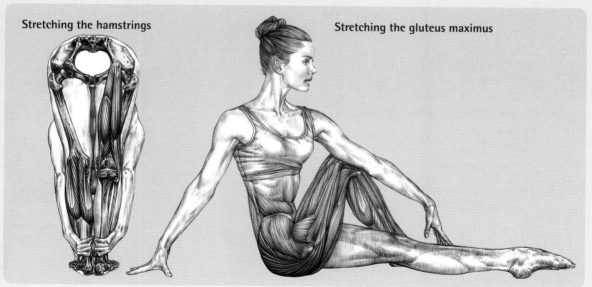

Stretching the hamstrings

Stretching the gluteus maximus

199

GAIN FLEXIBILITY IN THE ROTATOR MUSCLES OF THE HIPS

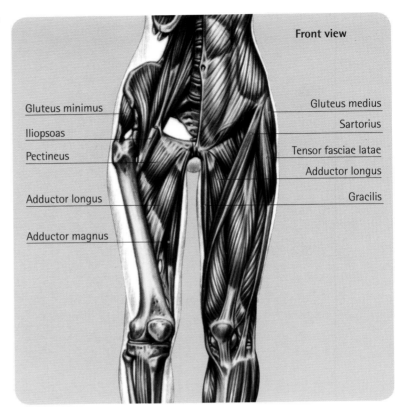

Front view

Gluteus minimus

Iliopsoas

Pectineus

Adductor longus

Adductor magnus

Gluteus medius

Sartorius

Tensor fasciae latae

Adductor longus

Gracilis

The rotator muscles of the hips have a very important role in maintaining the proper curve in the lumbar spine. When these muscles are not flexible enough, their stiffness pulls on the lower back, making the lumbar spine lose its natural curve. This misalignment makes the intervertebral discs very vulnerable to the jolts normally experienced while running or even when walking. Proper technique in sports that require hip rotation, such as golf, can be adversely affected by this stiffness. Athletes should therefore be mindful of the flexibility of these rotator muscles. The same is true for anyone wanting to avoid back problems. Most people experience these kinds of problems.

Strengthening the rotator muscles of the hips is particularly important for sports that are hard on the hips, such as soccer, martial arts, and golf. Developing these muscles is even more important because they are so often neglected.

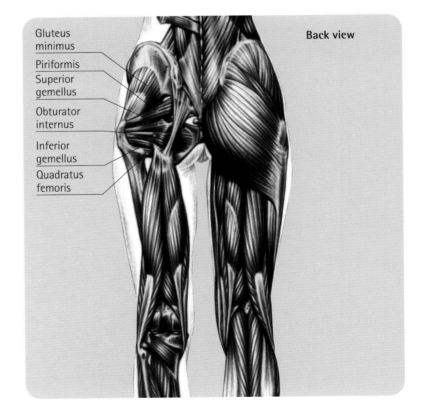

Back view

Gluteus minimus

Piriformis

Superior gemellus

Obturator internus

Inferior gemellus

Quadratus femoris

/// Checking the Rotator Muscles in the Hips

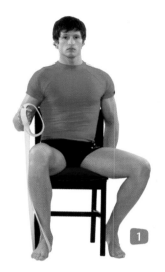 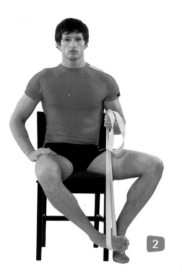 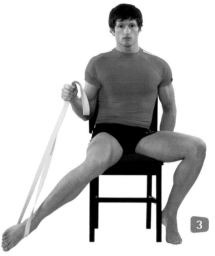

1 To check the flexibility in your hips, sit down on the highest chair you have. Ideally, your feet should not touch the floor.

2 Using a band (without forcing things), lift your right foot as high as you can toward your left side while keeping your leg bent to 90 degrees. Keep your thigh glued to the chair the entire time. Normal flexibility should permit a 45- to 65-degree rotation of the thigh.

3 Then, lift your right foot to the right. You should be able to move it 30 to 45 degrees.

Perform the same test on the left leg.

/// Stretching the Hips

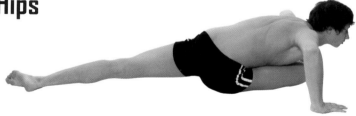

If you are not very flexible, you will need to do stretching exercises. There are three complementary stretches.

For the first two exercises, simply repeat the previous exercises, again using a band. Keep the other end of the band in your hand so you can work on the flexibility of the muscles by pulling lightly on the band. Work progressively and do not make any abrupt movements.

The third exercise is more complex. Sitting with the right leg crossed in front of you, lean your torso forward onto the right leg and stretch the left leg out behind you. Once you have stretched the right leg, repeat the stretch on the left leg.

To strengthen the rotator muscles, always use a band around your foot and hold the other end in your hand. Do the opposite movement of the two test exercises described above. Increase the resistance by pulling lightly on the band with your hand. Always work in long sets using continuous tension. Do not make any jerky or abrupt movements.

SCULPT YOUR ABDOMINALS

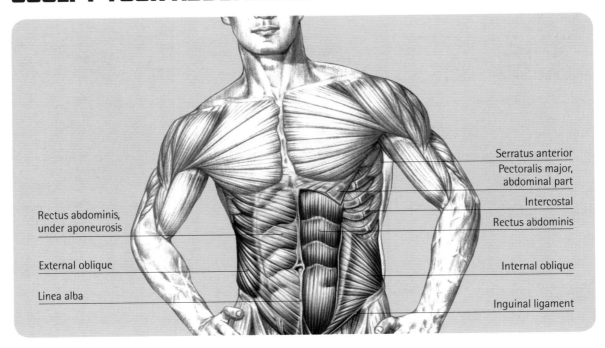

Serratus anterior

Pectoralis major, abdominal part

Intercostal

Rectus abdominis

Rectus abdominis, under aponeurosis

External oblique

Linea alba

Internal oblique

Inguinal ligament

▌Role of the Abdominal Muscles

The abdominal muscles have a very important role in protecting the spine. This is why they are fundamental in most sports and especially in weight training. They also support the respiratory muscles and the thighs during movement.

Aesthetically, the abdominal muscles are extremely important since they clearly reveal a lean physique. Chiseled abdominal muscles are a sign of virility in men. Strong abdominal muscles help keep the belly flat. In this task, they are assisted by the deep abdominal muscles.

Unfortunately, the lower-abdominal muscles are much more difficult to recruit and strengthen than the upper-abdominal muscles. It is possible to do bridges mostly with the strength of the upper-abdominal muscles. This is why bridge exercises are more complicated to master than crunches.

However, the lower-abdominal muscles play the biggest role in protecting the spine and warding off belly fat. This is where fat accumulates most easily. A good circuit for the abdominal muscles must therefore work not only the upper section but also the lower section.

Direction of abdominal muscles' movement and the system containing viscera

In humans, with the evolution to walking on two feet, the abdominal muscles were considerably strengthened to synchronize the movement of the pelvis with the torso while in a vertical position, preventing the torso from moving excessively during walking or running. They became powerful stabilizing muscles, actively sheathing the viscera.

1 Rectus abdominis
2 External oblique
3 Internal oblique
4 Transversus abdominis

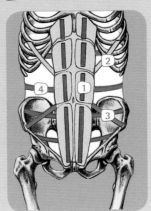

NOTE

The abdominal muscles work on both ends. Exercises that raise the torso recruit the upper-abdominal muscles (but not exclusively). Exercises that raise the lower part of the body target the lower-abdominal muscles a bit more.

Action of the abdominal muscles

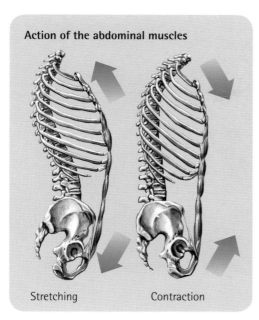

Stretching   Contraction

Abdominal muscles

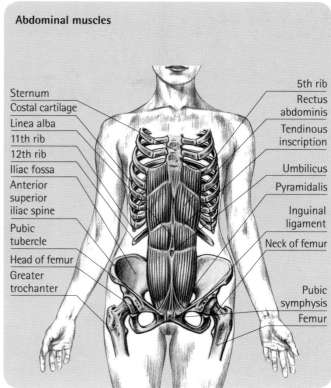

Sternum
Costal cartilage
Linea alba
11th rib
12th rib
Iliac fossa
Anterior superior iliac spine
Pubic tubercle
Head of femur
Greater trochanter

5th rib
Rectus abdominis
Tendinous inscription
Umbilicus
Pyramidalis
Inguinal ligament
Neck of femur
Pubic symphysis
Femur

Sections of various types of inner-abdominal walls

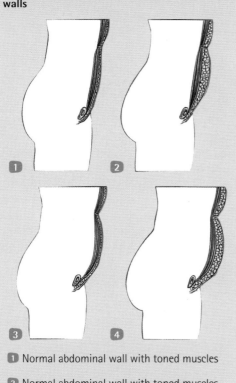

1 Normal abdominal wall with toned muscles

2 Normal abdominal wall with toned muscles and subcutaneous fat creating a bulge

3 Bulging abdominal wall with weak muscles and no fat

4 Bulging abdominal wall with weak muscles and a layer of fat

Deep abdominal muscles

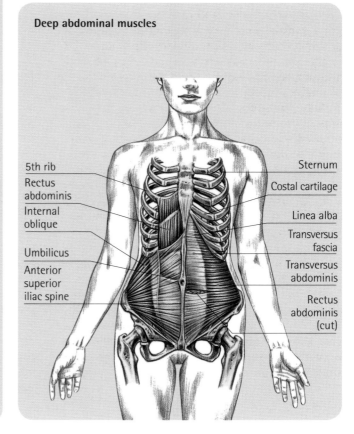

5th rib
Rectus abdominis
Internal oblique
Umbilicus
Anterior superior iliac spine

Sternum
Costal cartilage
Linea alba
Transversus fascia
Transversus abdominis
Rectus abdominis (cut)

Not all abdominal exercises are the same!

Several ineffective abdominal exercises can endanger the spine. There is an easy way to tell the good exercises from the bad. In a bad exercise, the lower back will arch when the abdominal muscles contract. Therefore, all exercises that arch the lumbar spine do not work the abdominal muscles effectively.

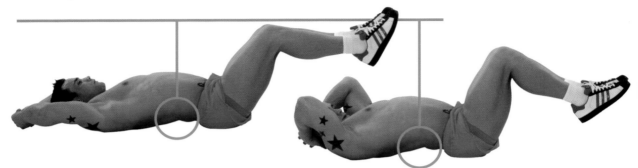

Pay attention to your head!

The position of your head has a profound impact on muscle contraction. When you lean your head back, the lumbar muscles supporting the spine contract reflexively while the abdominal muscles have a tendency to relax. Even if the contraction is not very intense, it is inevitable. However, when you tilt your head forward, the abdominal muscles contract and the lumbar muscles relax. The body has a tendency to arch forward. This is why if you are standing up and looking above you, you tend to fall backward. If you look down, you tend to fall forward.

ABDOMINALS

The muscles responsible for movement in ineffective and potentially dangerous abdominal exercises are the psoas major, iliacus, and rectus femoris. You will know they are involved as soon as an exercise forces you to arch your back. For example, exercises that involve putting your legs in the air for as long as possible and scissor movements while lying down are "back breakers." Since the abdominal muscles are attached to the pelvis and not to the thighs, they cannot make the legs move.

Why are these movements so painful? Since arching the back is dangerous for the lumbar discs, the abdominal muscles will try to intervene to straighten the spine. They contract isometrically (that is, without moving), which deprives them of oxygen since their local blood circulation is blocked. Large quantities of lactic acid then build up in the abdominal muscles since it cannot be removed because of poor blood circulation. This artificial asphyxiation causes an intense burning sensation. It is a bit like going for a jog with a bag on your head; you will not last very long. In addition, it is dangerous and counterproductive to good performance. Isometric contraction is not effective for developing the abdominal muscles or burning fat.

You also must define a clear strategy for the position of your head during a weight training exercise. What you must avoid is moving your head from side to side. These unhelpful movements interfere with proper muscle contraction and could cause problems in your cervical spine. Except in unilateral exercises, you should never turn your head to the side. And if your head is turned to the side, you should never move it during the exercise. In the same way, it is totally counterproductive to shake your head vigorously when the exercise gets really hard. This is when your body should work hard to avoid a lot of unnecessary movements.

During abdominal exercises, keep your head tilted forward and, above all, do not look at the ceiling. With your head in the air, the resulting reflex contraction will prevent the proper rolling of the body. When you work the abdominal muscles, you should always keep your eyes on your abdomen. However, when you do the squat, for example, keeping your head high helps your balance and protects the spine. If you move the head from left to right, the small reflex contractions that follow will alternatively recruit and then relax the muscles on the left and then the right sides. This will interfere with the proper execution of the exercise.

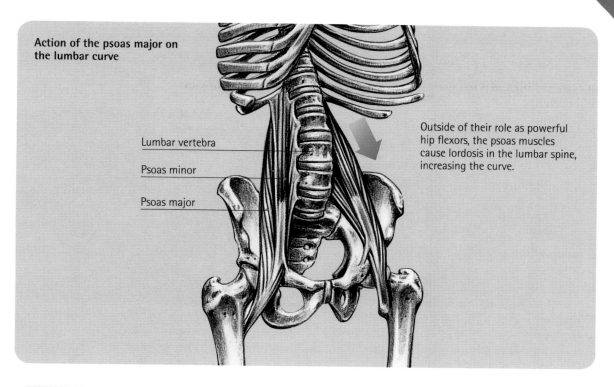

Action of the psoas major on the lumbar curve

Lumbar vertebra

Psoas minor

Psoas major

Outside of their role as powerful hip flexors, the psoas muscles cause lordosis in the lumbar spine, increasing the curve.

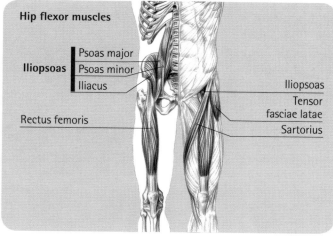

Hip flexor muscles

Iliopsoas
- Psoas major
- Psoas minor
- Iliacus

Rectus femoris

Iliopsoas

Tensor fasciae latae

Sartorius

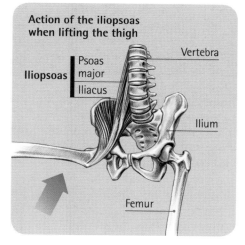

Action of the iliopsoas when lifting the thigh

Vertebra

Iliopsoas
- Psoas major
- Iliacus

Ilium

Femur

During abdominal exercises, it is important to round your spine. As with most abdominal exercises, never arch your back when doing leg lifts off the floor.

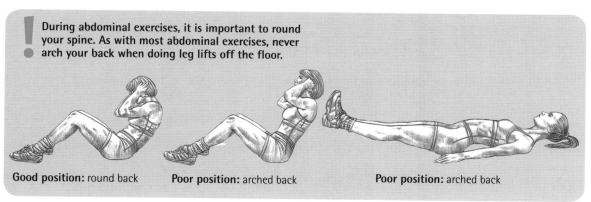

Good position: round back   **Poor position:** arched back   **Poor position:** arched back

/// Crunch

This is an isolation exercise for the entire abdominal area but primarily for the upper-abdominal muscles. Unilateral work is possible mainly for versions with side rotation.

> **NOTES**
> This exercise is especially good for sports where jumping and running are required.

> ! If you pull with your torso or with your hands behind your head to get up more easily, you could pinch your lumbar and cervical spine.

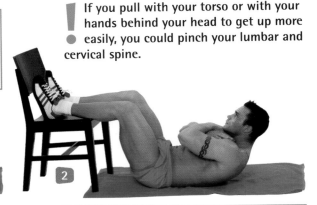

1 Lie on the floor with your legs bent or your feet on a chair. Cross your hands on your chest (left hand on the right shoulder and right hand on the left shoulder).

2 Rise up slowly without jerking to lift your shoulders and then your upper spine off the floor. Pause for two seconds in this position while strongly contracting your abdominal muscles. Return slowly to the starting position and begin the exercise again with a smooth movement.

Exhale when you contract the abdominal muscles. By emptying the lungs, you can increase the contraction. Breathe in while lowering your torso to the floor.

If you can do more than 20 repetitions, then you are not doing the exercise correctly. The most common error is not locking out the abdominal muscles at the top of the movement. The goal is not to do as many repetitions as possible but rather to contract the muscles as tightly as possible during each repetition.

HELPFUL HINTS

The position of your hands determines the difficulty of this exercise. We have described a standard neutral position in terms of resistance from the arms.

Stretching the arms along the body will make the exercise easier.

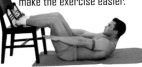

Putting your hands behind your head makes the exercise harder. One possible combination is to begin with your arms behind your head. At failure, stretch your arms out in front so that you can do a few more repetitions.

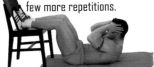

You can use a weight plate to increase the resistance.

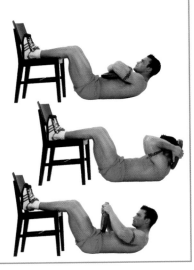

ADVANTAGES

Crunches are simple exercises that really work the abdominal muscles without endangering the spine.

- - - - - - - - - - - - - - - - - - - -

The range of motion in crunches is rather small (6 inches, or 15 cm). It is tempting to try to increase the range of motion by lifting the entire torso off the floor. In this case, the abdominal work becomes secondary, and you put the integrity of your spine in jeopardy.

DISADVANTAGES

ABDOMINALS

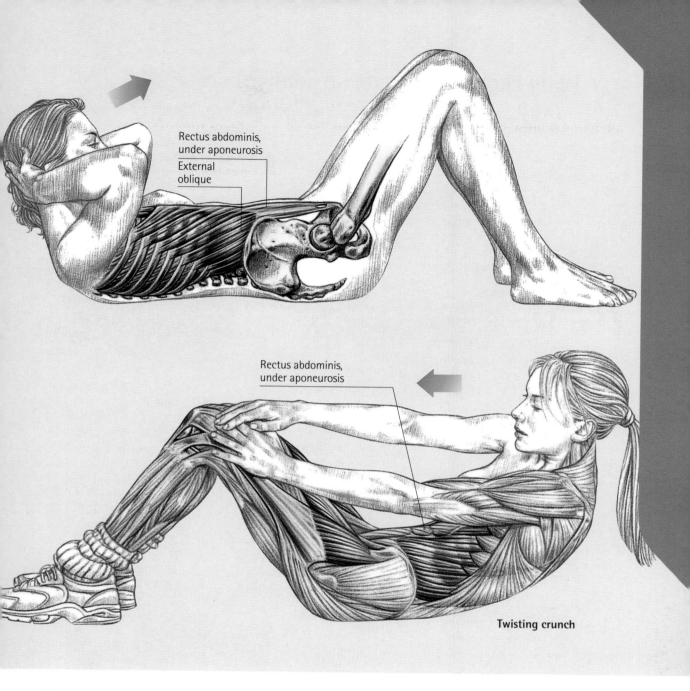

Rectus abdominis,
under aponeurosis

External
oblique

Rectus abdominis,
under aponeurosis

Twisting crunch

(**Variations**)

To work the oblique muscles a little more when you are working the abdominal muscles, you can rotate your torso to the side instead of coming straight up.

To work the left side, put your right hand behind your head and place your left arm out to the side on the floor so it serves as a pivot.

This will facilitate the side rotation. Without using jerky movements, bring your right elbow toward your left thigh using the strength of your abdominal muscles. The goal is not to touch your thigh with your elbow, because the movement generally stops halfway. Hold the position for two seconds before lowering

your torso. To maintain continuous tension, do not rest your head on the floor. Once you have finished on the right side, repeat the exercise on the left side. Again, stretching the arms along the body makes the exercise easier, and putting both hands behind the head makes the exercise harder.

/// Lying Leg Raise (Reverse Crunch)

This is an isolation exercise for the entire abdominal area but primarily for the lower-abdominal muscles. Unilateral work is possible but not desirable because it tends to compress the spine.

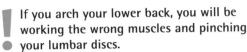

! If you arch your lower back, you will be working the wrong muscles and pinching your lumbar discs.

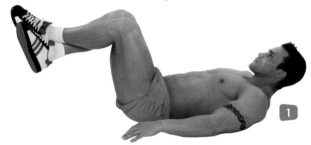

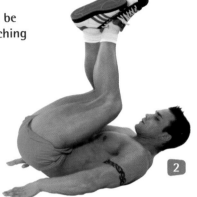

1 Lie on the floor with your arms at your sides and your legs bent to 90 degrees.

2 Lift up your buttocks and then your lower back by rolling the opposite way that you would for a crunch. You must roll slowly, stopping when you feel your upper back starting to come off the floor. Try to bring your lower-abdominal muscles up to touch your pectoralis muscles. They should not actually touch, but by concentrating on this imaginary goal, you will achieve the correct movement. Pause for at least two seconds in the upper position while deeply contracting your abdominal muscles.

3 Return slowly to the starting position and stop before your buttocks touch the floor in order to maintain continuous tension. Keep your head very straight on the floor. Do not move your neck.

ABDOMINALS

ADVANTAGES

The lower-abdominal muscle is the most difficult part of the muscle to work. Leg raises are the main exercise that will teach you to work the lower part of the muscle.

- -

It is easier to do this exercise poorly than it is to do it well. A pulling sensation in the lower spine means you are doing the exercise incorrectly. It will take some time to learn this exercise so that you will know how to contract the lower part of your abdominal muscles tightly.

DISADVANTAGES

HELPFUL HINTS
The goal of this exercise is not so much to lift your legs. The goal is to lift your hips, which will lift the thighs, but the thighs always stay in the same position.

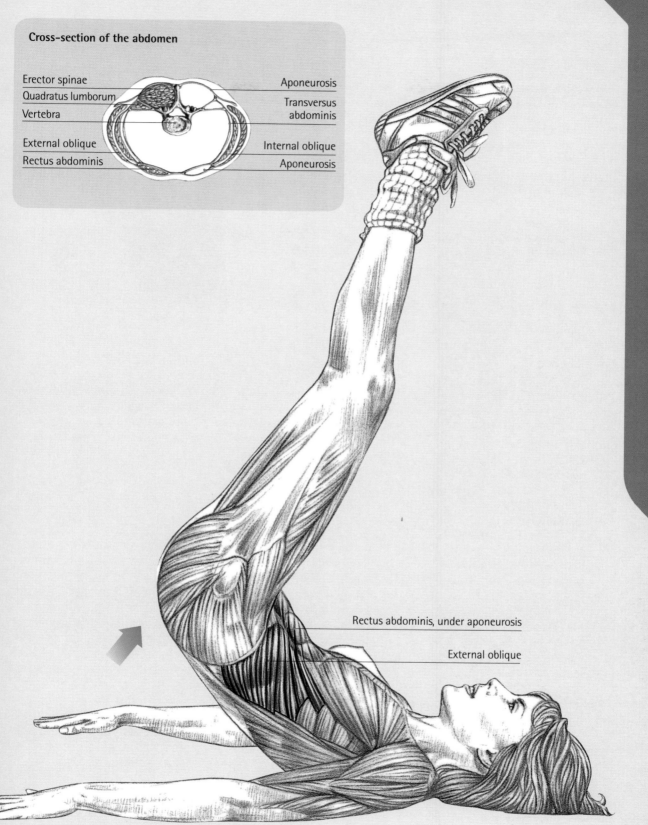

Cross-section of the abdomen

Erector spinae

Quadratus lumborum

Vertebra

External oblique

Rectus abdominis

Aponeurosis

Transversus abdominis

Internal oblique

Aponeurosis

Rectus abdominis, under aponeurosis

External oblique

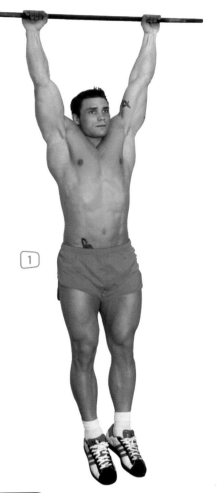

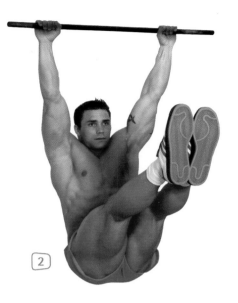

Variations

Keeping your legs straight throughout the movement makes the exercise easier to do. The exercise is harder if you bend your legs so the calves touch the backs of the thighs. A good combination is to begin with bent legs, and at failure, straighten your legs and do a few more repetitions.

1 To make the exercise even harder, you can do it while hanging from a pull-up bar. Hang onto the bar with pronated hands (thumbs facing each other) about shoulder-width apart. Bring your legs to 90 degrees in relation to your torso so that your thighs are parallel to the floor. You can keep your legs straight (this makes the exercise a lot more difficult) or bring your calves under your thighs (this makes the exercise easier).

2 Using your lower-abdominal muscles, move your pelvis up while bringing your knees up toward your chest. Lift your pelvis as high as possible while rolling yourself up as much as you can. Hold the position for one second before lowering the pelvis. Be careful not to lower your legs past the point where they are parallel to the floor.

The hardest thing about this exercise when you first try it is to avoid moving too much. As you train more, you will learn to stabilize yourself naturally.

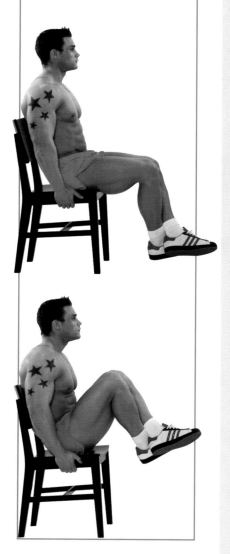

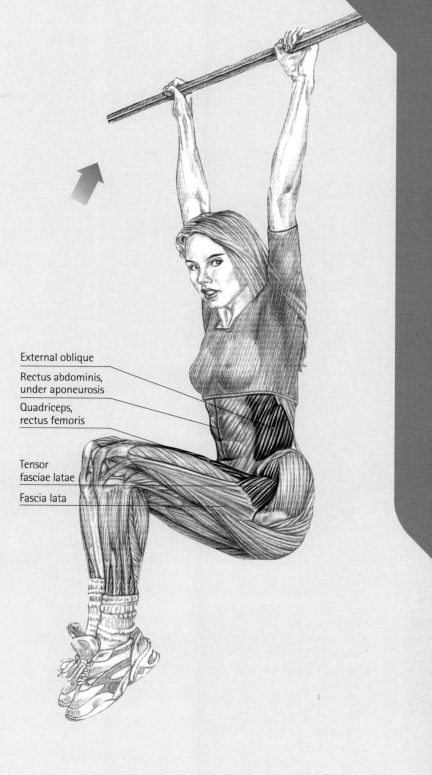

External oblique

Rectus abdominis, under aponeurosis

Quadriceps, rectus femoris

Tensor fasciae latae

Fascia lata

Obliques

The oblique muscles are located on both sides of the abdomen. They support the spine and have a major role in rotating the pelvis.

> ! If you arch your lower back, you will work the wrong muscles and pinch your lumbar discs.

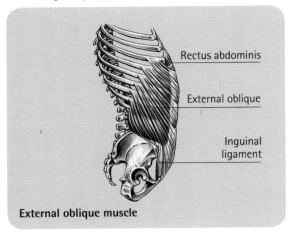

External oblique muscle

Rectus abdominis

External oblique

Inguinal ligament

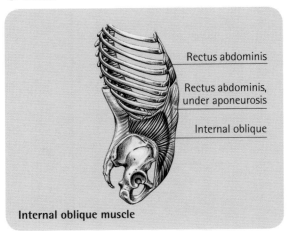

Internal oblique muscle

Rectus abdominis

Rectus abdominis, under aponeurosis

Internal oblique

/// Side Crunch

This is an isolation exercise for the oblique muscles. It must be done unilaterally.

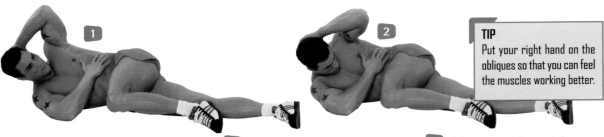

TIP
Put your right hand on the obliques so that you can feel the muscles working better.

1 Lie on your right side on the floor or on a bed. Put your left hand behind your head to support it. Bend your left leg to 90 degrees and keep your right leg semistraight. Push gently on your right knee with your left foot to increase your stability.

2 Using your obliques, bring your left elbow toward your right hip. Your right elbow will come off the floor about an inch or so. Hold the position for one to two seconds before lowering your torso. Bring your right shoulder to the floor, but not your head, so you can maintain continuous tension in your obliques. Once you have finished a set on the left side, move immediately to your right side.

ADVANTAGES

This is the perfect exercise for working the obliques. If you do the exercise correctly, you will feel your muscles working right away.

Unless it is required for a strength sport, you should not use too heavy a weight when working your obliques. Heavy weights increase the size of the muscles, but large obliques do not look very good. Instead, use light weights and do long sets so you can accentuate their definition and eliminate the fat that easily accumulates there.

DISADVANTAGES

HELPFUL HINTS
Do not do this exercise in a straight line. You should rotate your torso slightly from back to front while contracting your obliques.

NOTES
It is better to end your abdominal workout with the obliques rather than begin with them. Your priority should be the abdominal muscles and not the obliques.

ABDOMINALS

212

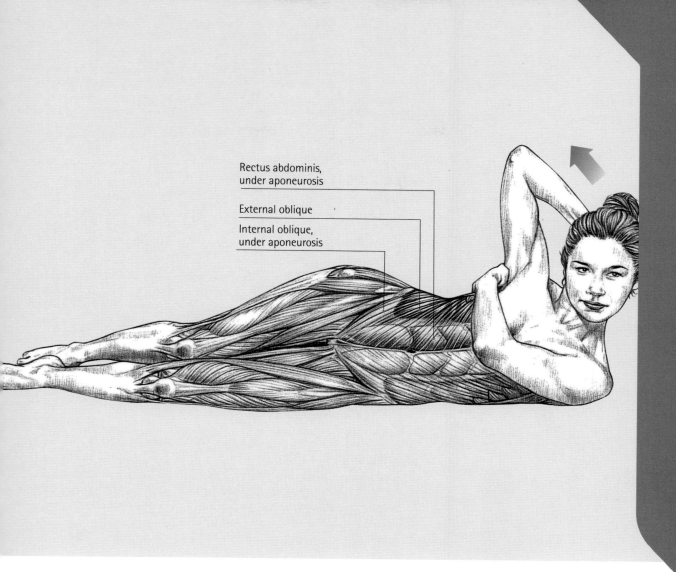

Rectus abdominis,
under aponeurosis

External oblique

Internal oblique,
under aponeurosis

! Do not make jerky move-
ments with your head so
that you can do a few more
repetitions, because that will
endanger your cervical spine.

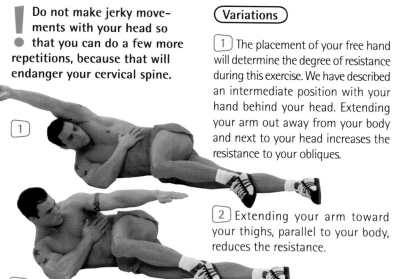

1

2

Variations

1 The placement of your free hand
will determine the degree of resistance
during this exercise. We have described
an intermediate position with your
hand behind your head. Extending
your arm out away from your body
and next to your head increases the
resistance to your obliques.

2 Extending your arm toward
your thighs, parallel to your body,
reduces the resistance.

A good combination is to begin
the exercise with your arm straight
up by your head, and at failure, put
your hand behind your head so that
you can do a few more repetitions.
When you reach failure again, stretch
your arm down toward your legs so
you can continue the exercise. You
can also do a few forced repetitions
by grabbing the upper-back part
of your thigh with your free hand.
Use your arm to pull your torso and
reduce the work on your obliques.
You should use this strategy only at
the end of a set. Your goal is to wear
out your obliques so that you will
not need to do as many sets.

/// Standing Twist

This is an isolation exercise for the obliques. It attacks the love handles better than any other exercise. It must be done unilaterally to create significant resistance on the muscles.

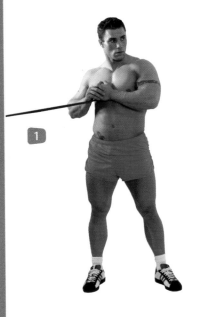

1 Attach a band to a fixed point at about shoulder height. Stand up and grab the band in both hands. Take a step forward. The farther away you move from the point where the band is attached, the greater the resistance you create.

2 Separate your legs to increase your stability and begin rotating from the right to the left. Do not turn your torso more than 45 degrees. When you have finished working the right side, move to the left side without pausing in between.

ADVANTAGES

Very few exercises target the love handles. Even so, love handles are not easy to eliminate. Only proper diet plus specific exercises will improve your chance of getting rid of them.

If you have back problems, do not do this exercise.

DISADVANTAGES

HELPFUL HINTS

This exercise is valuable only if there is lateral resistance. Frantically twisting from side to side with a weight bar on the shoulders as you so often see people do serves no purpose except to wear down the spine. The wear on the lumbar discs is even worse if you have a weighted bar on your shoulders.

NOTES

You should do this exercise slowly in long sets (25 repetitions). You can do two to four sets every day to combat love handles.

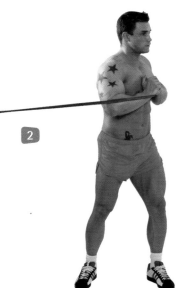

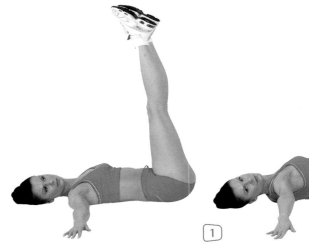

ABDOMINALS

(**Variations**)

1 You can also do twists on the floor with bent legs or straight legs (straight legs are the more difficult version).

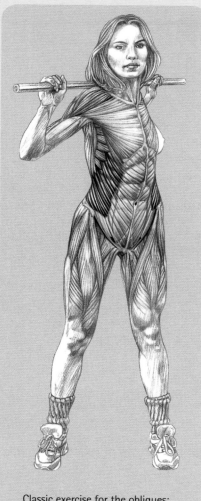

Classic exercise for the obliques:
dangerous and not effective

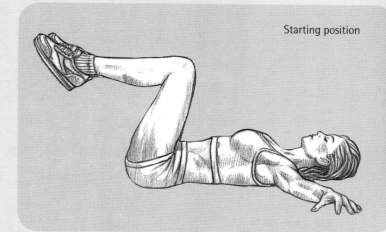

Starting position

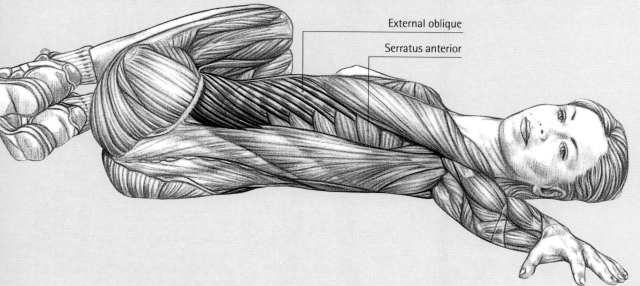

External oblique

Serratus anterior

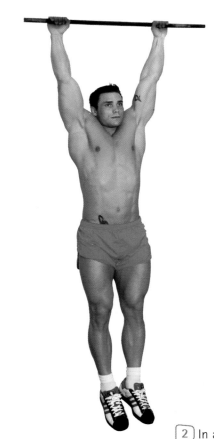

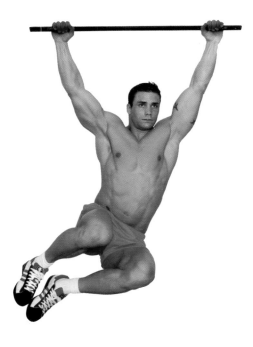

[2]

[2] In addition, twists (with bent legs or straight legs) can be done at the pull-up bar. This version also has the advantage of decompressing the spine at the end of a workout.

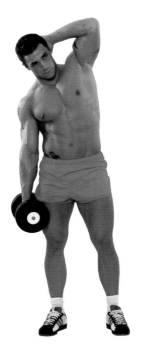

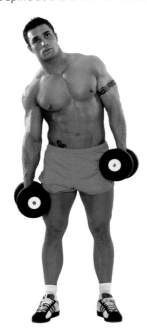

! Do not turn too far or too fast. Try to do a good contraction slowly over a short range of motion rather than an explosive movement with maximum range of motion. Be careful when doing side work on the obliques using dumbbells. These exercises are useful only in strength sports where enormous pressure is applied to the spine.

Above all, avoid using two dumbbells at the same time. This movement should be done only unilaterally.

Exercises for the Diaphragm and Respiratory Muscles

▌Respiratory Muscles and Endurance

Scientific research has shown that, during endurance work, the respiratory muscles, especially the diaphragm, get tired. As with other muscles, this fatigue decreases performance. However, weight training exercises for the diaphragm cause a notable improvement in endurance. Well-trained athletes also have larger diaphragms than sedentary people. Working the abdominal muscles in long sets will also help reduce breathlessness during a prolonged effort.

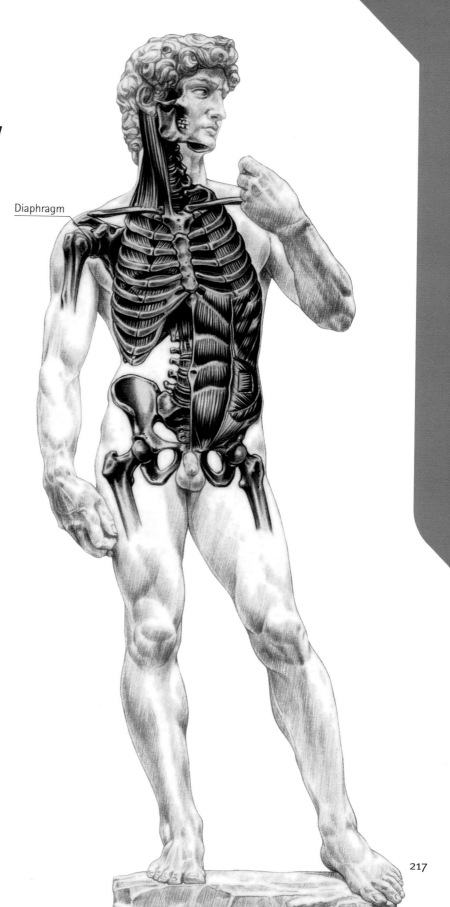

Diaphragm

217

/// Diaphragm Contraction

This is an exercise for the diaphragm as well as for the respiratory muscles.

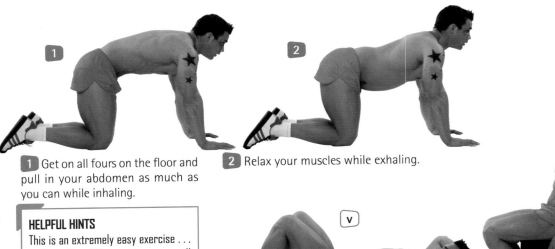

1 Get on all fours on the floor and pull in your abdomen as much as you can while inhaling.

2 Relax your muscles while exhaling.

HELPFUL HINTS
This is an extremely easy exercise . . . at first. After 20 repetitions, you will feel an unusual fatigue. This is when strengthening begins. Do as many repetitions as possible!

NOTES
During heavy exercises such as deadlifts or squats, the diaphragm is activated to increase intrathoracic pressure to protect the back. During weight training exercises that seriously compress the spine, strengthening the diaphragm might be necessary for people who have back problems.

Variations

v If you have trouble doing this exercise, you can do it sitting up (which is a little easier) or lying on your back (which is even easier).

To gain the most endurance, you can do the following superset:

> Begin on all fours until you tire out the respiratory muscles.

> At failure, turn over on your back so you can continue doing the easier version of the exercise.

ADVANTAGES
This exercise also works the transversus abdominis muscles—the ones that help keep your abdomen flat.

/// Rib Cage Expansion

By making thoracic expansion more difficult, **this exercise strengthens the muscles used during inhalation.**

HELPFUL HINTS
This exercise is useful only if it is done in long sets (at least 50 repetitions).

Lie on the floor and put a weight plate on your chest. Take a deep breath in so that you expand your rib cage fully. Exhale completely to deflate the rib cage.

Variations

To strengthen the respiratory muscles, you can also use resistance against the inflation of the rib cage in the form of an elastic sheath that lightly squeezes the chest during endurance exercises.

! **Do not begin with a heavy weight that will cave in your ribs. Begin with a light weight so that you can get your rib cage used to this exercise.**

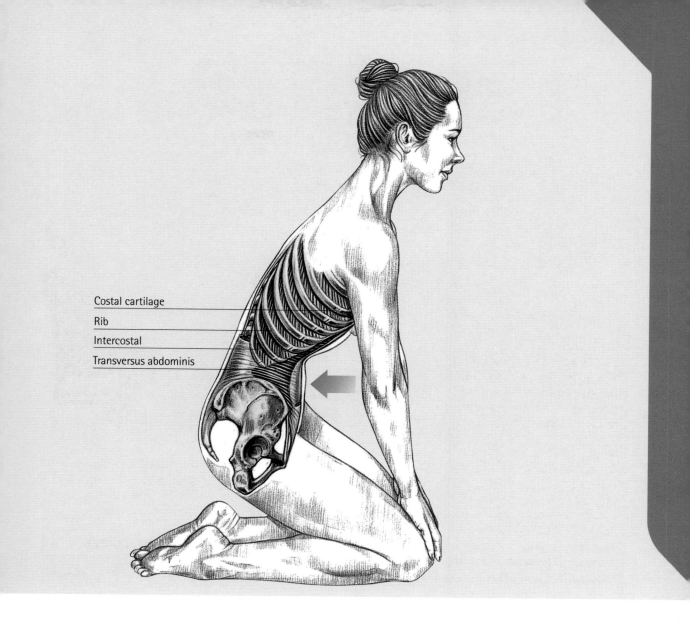

Costal cartilage

Rib

Intercostal

Transversus abdominis

/// Should You Stretch Your Abdominal Muscles?

To maintain a flat belly, we advise you not to stretch your abdominal muscles too much. Do not overdo the following stretch either with too many repetitions or too great a range of motion.

However, it is important to ensure flexibility in the psoas and iliacus muscles. This stretch occurs during lunges when you keep your torso very straight (described in the section on the thighs; see page 160).

Programming

Men's Strength

Know How to Focus Your Muscle Work to Save Time

The ideal is, of course, to work all of your muscles. However, to appear muscular, it is enough just to focus on a few key muscles. This first program for quickly gaining muscle mass highlights these key areas. By focusing on increasing muscle mass, you can achieve an impressive visual effect in an accelerated time frame.

The other advantage of focusing on key muscles is that it is possible to obtain a good physique, even if you do not have a lot of time to work out. Following are the key muscles:

> Lateral part of the shoulders (which creates the build)
> Exterior part of the triceps (which accentuates the size)
> Biceps (which give you big arms)
> Pectoralis muscles (which help define the torso)
> Abdominal muscles (which, when well defined, ensure a small, flat waist)

The back muscles are not highly visible, so they do not receive priority training. The same goes for the thighs and the calves.

> **NOTE**
> When you begin weight training, choose the lowest number of sets indicated. After several weeks of working out, slowly increase the number of sets so that you eventually reach the higher number.
> In the case of tapering sets, the higher number of repetitions indicated shows what you must do before starting to taper to a lower range at an increased weight. After that, do your maximum.

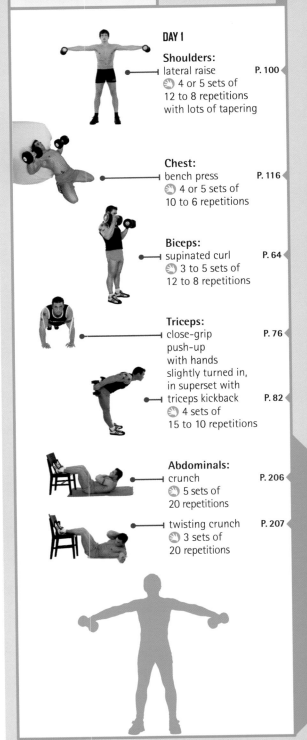

Beginner Program for Quickly Gaining Muscle Mass: Two Days per Week

DAY 1

Shoulders:
lateral raise — P. 100
4 or 5 sets of 12 to 8 repetitions with lots of tapering

Chest:
bench press — P. 116
4 or 5 sets of 10 to 6 repetitions

Biceps:
supinated curl — P. 64
3 to 5 sets of 12 to 8 repetitions

Triceps:
close-grip push-up with hands slightly turned in, in superset with — P. 76
triceps kickback — P. 82
4 sets of 15 to 10 repetitions

Abdominals:
crunch — P. 206
5 sets of 20 repetitions

twisting crunch — P. 207
3 sets of 20 repetitions

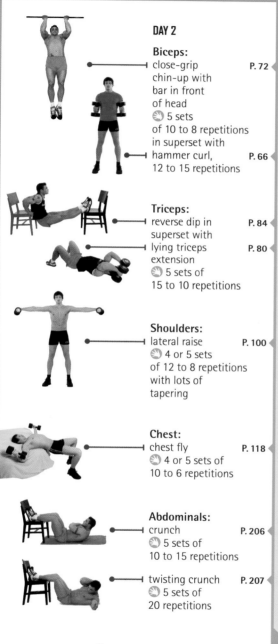

DAY 2

Biceps:
close-grip chin-up with bar in front of head   P. 72
5 sets of 10 to 8 repetitions in superset with
hammer curl,   P. 66
12 to 15 repetitions

Triceps:
reverse dip in superset with   P. 84
lying triceps extension   P. 80
5 sets of 15 to 10 repetitions

Shoulders:
lateral raise   P. 100
4 or 5 sets of 12 to 8 repetitions with lots of tapering

Chest:
chest fly   P. 118
4 or 5 sets of 10 to 6 repetitions

Abdominals:
crunch   P. 206
5 sets of 10 to 15 repetitions

twisting crunch   P. 207
5 sets of 20 repetitions

Beginner Program for Quickly Gaining Muscle Mass:
Three Days per Week

If you are able to train three days a week and if you feel that you are in good shape, add in the following workout between the two workouts just described. It will complete the work that you do in your two regular workouts. However, you are not required to include it every week.

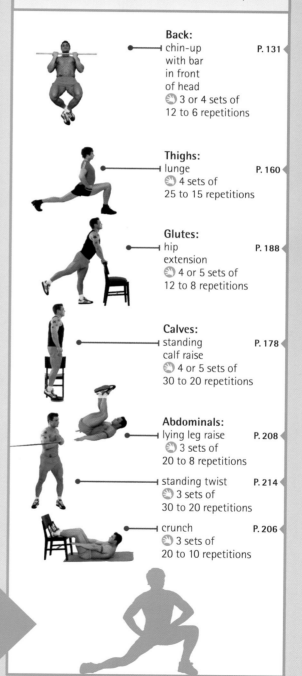

Back:
chin-up with bar in front of head   P. 131
3 or 4 sets of 12 to 6 repetitions

Thighs:
lunge   P. 160
4 sets of 25 to 15 repetitions

Glutes:
hip extension   P. 188
4 or 5 sets of 12 to 8 repetitions

Calves:
standing calf raise   P. 178
4 or 5 sets of 30 to 20 repetitions

Abdominals:
lying leg raise   P. 208
3 sets of 20 to 8 repetitions

standing twist   P. 214
3 sets of 30 to 20 repetitions

crunch   P. 206
3 sets of 20 to 10 repetitions

Advanced Program for Quickly Gaining Muscle Mass:
Three Days per Week

After doing the preceding program for one or two months, you can move on to a more advanced program so that you can continue to make progress.

If you feel the transition is too tiring, reduce the workload by one or two sets for each muscle group. When you feel ready, you can increase the number of sets.

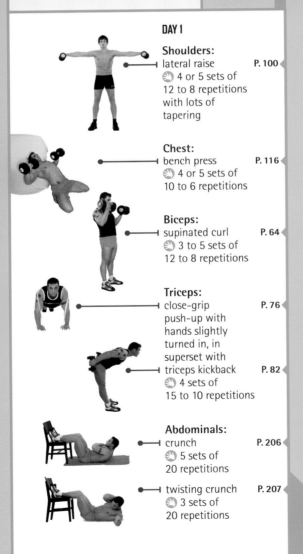

DAY 1

Shoulders:
lateral raise   **P. 100**
4 or 5 sets of 12 to 8 repetitions with lots of tapering

Chest:
bench press   **P. 116**
4 or 5 sets of 10 to 6 repetitions

Biceps:
supinated curl   **P. 64**
3 to 5 sets of 12 to 8 repetitions

Triceps:
close-grip push-up with hands slightly turned in, in superset with   **P. 76**

triceps kickback   **P. 82**
4 sets of 15 to 10 repetitions

Abdominals:
crunch   **P. 206**
5 sets of 20 repetitions

twisting crunch   **P. 207**
3 sets of 20 repetitions

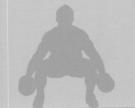

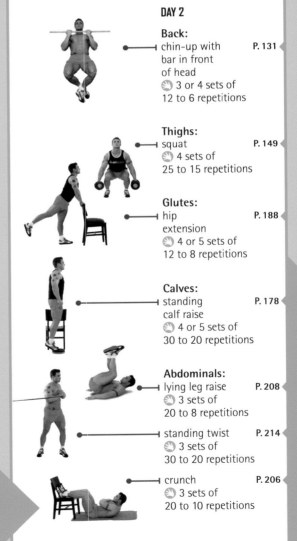

DAY 2

Back:
chin-up with bar in front of head   **P. 131**
3 or 4 sets of 12 to 6 repetitions

Thighs:
squat   **P. 149**
4 sets of 25 to 15 repetitions

Glutes:
hip extension   **P. 188**
4 or 5 sets of 12 to 8 repetitions

Calves:
standing calf raise   **P. 178**
4 or 5 sets of 30 to 20 repetitions

Abdominals:
lying leg raise   **P. 208**
3 sets of 20 to 8 repetitions

standing twist   **P. 214**
3 sets of 30 to 20 repetitions

crunch   **P. 206**
3 sets of 20 to 10 repetitions

After several months of training, you should be able to substitute more exercises from the ones in the second part of this book. This will help you to adapt the program better to your own needs and goals. You should also include some of your favorite techniques for increasing intensity.

Complete Strength Training Program for Beginners:
Two Days per Week

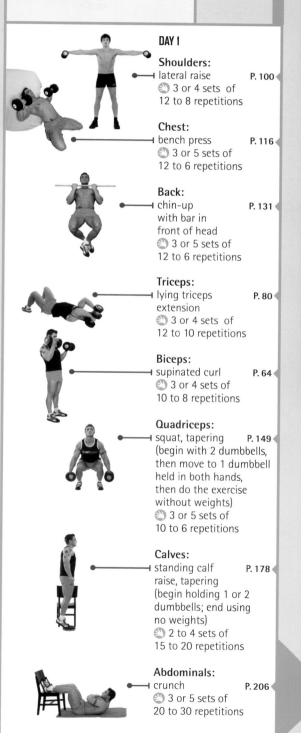

DAY 1

Shoulders:
lateral raise — P. 100
🕐 3 or 4 sets of 12 to 8 repetitions

Chest:
bench press — P. 116
🕐 3 or 5 sets of 12 to 6 repetitions

Back:
chin-up with bar in front of head — P. 131
🕐 3 or 5 sets of 12 to 6 repetitions

Triceps:
lying triceps extension — P. 80
🕐 3 or 4 sets of 12 to 10 repetitions

Biceps:
supinated curl — P. 64
🕐 3 or 4 sets of 10 to 8 repetitions

Quadriceps:
squat, tapering — P. 149
(begin with 2 dumbbells, then move to 1 dumbbell held in both hands, then do the exercise without weights)
🕐 3 or 5 sets of 10 to 6 repetitions

Calves:
standing calf raise, tapering — P. 178
(begin holding 1 or 2 dumbbells; end using no weights)
🕐 2 to 4 sets of 15 to 20 repetitions

Abdominals:
crunch — P. 206
🕐 3 or 5 sets of 20 to 30 repetitions

DAY 3

Biceps:
close-grip chin-up — P. 72

🕐 5 sets of 10 to 8 repetitions in superset with hammer curl, — P. 66
12 to 15 repetitions

Triceps:
reverse dip in — P. 84
superset with lying triceps extension — P. 80
🕐 5 sets of 15 to 10 repetitions

Shoulders:
lateral raise — P. 100
🕐 4 or 5 sets of 12 to 8 repetitions with lots of tapering

Chest:
chest fly — P. 118
🕐 4 or 5 sets of 10 to 6 repetitions

Abdominals:
crunch — P. 206
🕐 5 sets of 10 to 15 repetitions

twisting crunch — P. 207
🕐 3 sets of 20 repetitions

225

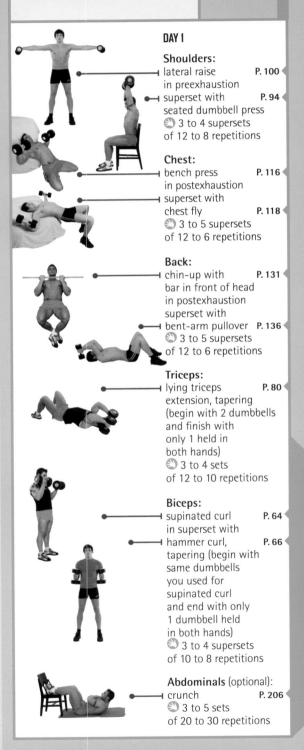

2

1

DAY 2

Chest:
push-up   P. 113
4 or 5 sets
of 12 to 6 repetitions

Back:
row   P. 134
3 to 5 sets
of 12 to 6 repetitions

Shoulders:
seated dumbbell   P. 94
press in
superset with
bent-over   P. 104
lateral raise
3 to 5 supersets
of 10 to 6 repetitions

Biceps:
supinated curl   P. 64
3 to 4 sets
of 12 to 10 repetitions

Triceps:
lying triceps   P. 80
extension
3 to 5 sets
of 12 to 6 repetitions

Hamstrings:
bent-legged   P. 143
deadlift
3 to 5 sets
of 12 to 6 repetitions

Quadriceps:
leg extension   P. 166
4 to 6 sets
of 10 to 6 repetitions

Calves:
donkey calf raise   P. 181
2 to 4 sets
of 25 to 50 repetitions

Abdominals: P. 210
leg raise
on pull-up
bar
3 to 5 sets
of 10 to 12 repetitions

DAY 1

Shoulders:
lateral raise   P. 100
in preexhaustion
superset with   P. 94
seated dumbbell press
3 to 4 supersets
of 12 to 8 repetitions

Chest:
bench press   P. 116
in postexhaustion
superset with
chest fly   P. 118
3 to 5 supersets
of 12 to 6 repetitions

Back:
chin-up with   P. 131
bar in front of head
in postexhaustion
superset with
bent-arm pullover   P. 136
3 to 5 supersets
of 12 to 6 repetitions

Triceps:
lying triceps   P. 80
extension, tapering
(begin with 2 dumbbells
and finish with
only 1 held in
both hands)
3 to 4 sets
of 12 to 10 repetitions

Biceps:
supinated curl   P. 64
in superset with
hammer curl,   P. 66
tapering (begin with
same dumbbells
you used for
supinated curl
and end with only
1 dumbbell held
in both hands)
3 to 4 supersets
of 10 to 8 repetitions

Abdominals (optional):
crunch   P. 206
3 to 5 sets
of 20 to 30 repetitions

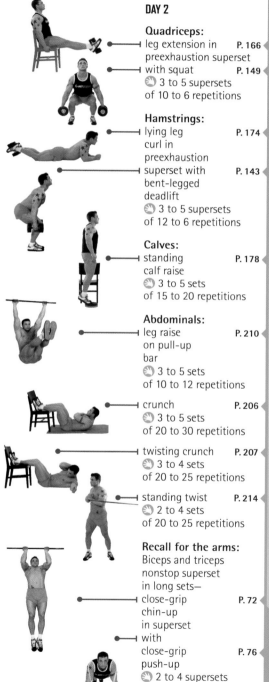

DAY 2

Quadriceps:
leg extension in
preexhaustion superset
with squat
P. 166
P. 149
🕑 3 to 5 supersets
of 10 to 6 repetitions

Hamstrings:
lying leg
curl in
preexhaustion
superset with
bent-legged
deadlift
P. 174
P. 143
🕑 3 to 5 supersets
of 12 to 6 repetitions

Calves:
standing
calf raise
P. 178
🕑 3 to 5 sets
of 15 to 20 repetitions

Abdominals:
leg raise
on pull-up
bar
P. 210
🕑 3 to 5 sets
of 10 to 12 repetitions

crunch
P. 206
🕑 3 to 5 sets
of 20 to 30 repetitions

twisting crunch
P. 207
🕑 3 to 4 sets
of 20 to 25 repetitions

standing twist
P. 214
🕑 2 to 4 sets
of 20 to 25 repetitions

Recall for the arms:
Biceps and triceps
nonstop superset
in long sets—
close-grip
chin-up
in superset
P. 72
with
close-grip
push-up
P. 76
🕑 2 to 4 supersets
of 12 to 6 repetitions

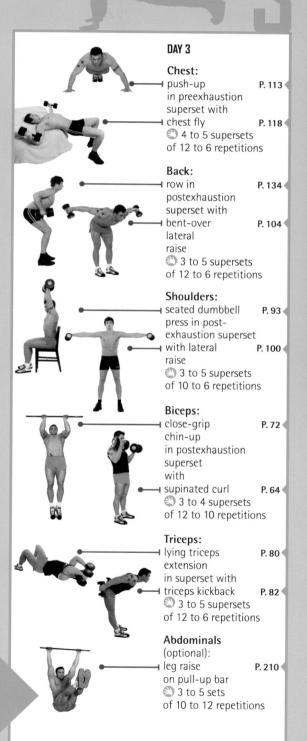

DAY 3

Chest:
push-up
in preexhaustion
superset with
chest fly
P. 113
P. 118
🕑 4 to 5 supersets
of 12 to 6 repetitions

Back:
row in
postexhaustion
superset with
bent-over
lateral
raise
P. 134
P. 104
🕑 3 to 5 supersets
of 12 to 6 repetitions

Shoulders:
seated dumbbell
press in post-
exhaustion superset
with lateral
raise
P. 93
P. 100
🕑 3 to 5 supersets
of 10 to 6 repetitions

Biceps:
close-grip
chin-up
in postexhaustion
superset
with
supinated curl
P. 72
P. 64
🕑 3 to 4 supersets
of 12 to 10 repetitions

Triceps:
lying triceps
extension
in superset with
triceps kickback
P. 80
P. 82
🕑 3 to 5 supersets
of 12 to 6 repetitions

Abdominals
(optional):
leg raise
on pull-up bar
P. 210
🕑 3 to 5 sets
of 10 to 12 repetitions

Advanced Complete Strength Training Program: Four Days per Week

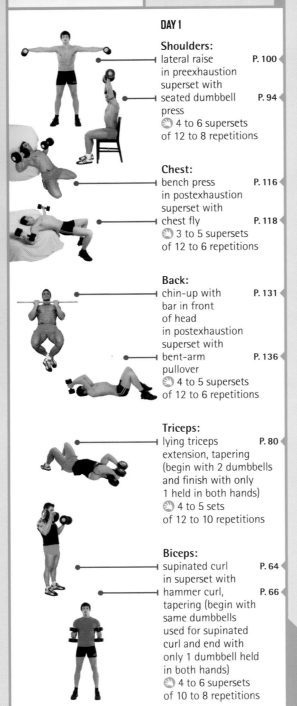

DAY 1

Shoulders:
lateral raise   P. 100
in preexhaustion
superset with
seated dumbbell   P. 94
press
4 to 6 supersets
of 12 to 8 repetitions

Chest:
bench press   P. 116
in postexhaustion
superset with
chest fly   P. 118
3 to 5 supersets
of 12 to 6 repetitions

Back:
chin-up with   P. 131
bar in front
of head
in postexhaustion
superset with
bent-arm   P. 136
pullover
4 to 5 supersets
of 12 to 6 repetitions

Triceps:
lying triceps   P. 80
extension, tapering
(begin with 2 dumbbells
and finish with only
1 held in both hands)
4 to 5 sets
of 12 to 10 repetitions

Biceps:
supinated curl   P. 64
in superset with
hammer curl,   P. 66
tapering (begin with
same dumbbells
used for supinated
curl and end with
only 1 dumbbell held
in both hands)
4 to 6 supersets
of 10 to 8 repetitions

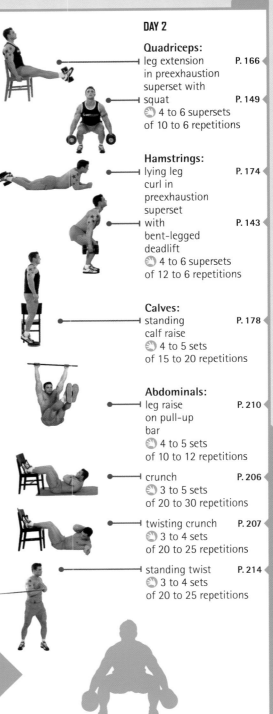

DAY 2

Quadriceps:
leg extension   P. 166
in preexhaustion
superset with
squat   P. 149
4 to 6 supersets
of 10 to 6 repetitions

Hamstrings:
lying leg   P. 174
curl in
preexhaustion
superset
with   P. 143
bent-legged
deadlift
4 to 6 supersets
of 12 to 6 repetitions

Calves:
standing   P. 178
calf raise
4 to 5 sets
of 15 to 20 repetitions

Abdominals:
leg raise   P. 210
on pull-up
bar
4 to 5 sets
of 10 to 12 repetitions

crunch   P. 206
3 to 5 sets
of 20 to 30 repetitions

twisting crunch   P. 207
3 to 4 sets
of 20 to 25 repetitions

standing twist   P. 214
3 to 4 sets
of 20 to 25 repetitions

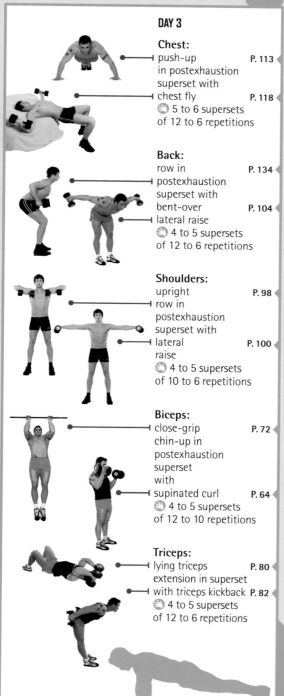

DAY 3

Chest:
push-up   P. 113
in postexhaustion
superset with
chest fly   P. 118
5 to 6 supersets
of 12 to 6 repetitions

Back:
row in   P. 134
postexhaustion
superset with
bent-over
lateral raise   P. 104
4 to 5 supersets
of 12 to 6 repetitions

Shoulders:
upright   P. 98
row in
postexhaustion
superset with
lateral   P. 100
raise
4 to 5 supersets
of 10 to 6 repetitions

Biceps:
close-grip   P. 72
chin-up in
postexhaustion
superset
with
supinated curl   P. 64
4 to 5 supersets
of 12 to 10 repetitions

Triceps:
lying triceps   P. 80
extension in superset
with triceps kickback   P. 82
4 to 5 supersets
of 12 to 6 repetitions

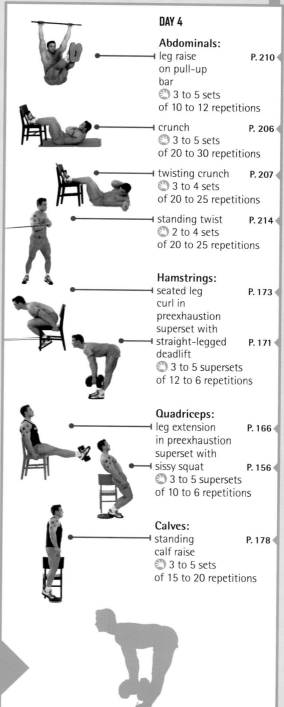

DAY 4

Abdominals:
leg raise   P. 210
on pull-up
bar
3 to 5 sets
of 10 to 12 repetitions

crunch   P. 206
3 to 5 sets
of 20 to 30 repetitions

twisting crunch   P. 207
3 to 4 sets
of 20 to 25 repetitions

standing twist   P. 214
2 to 4 sets
of 20 to 25 repetitions

Hamstrings:
seated leg   P. 173
curl in
preexhaustion
superset with
straight-legged   P. 171
deadlift
3 to 5 supersets
of 12 to 6 repetitions

Quadriceps:
leg extension   P. 166
in preexhaustion
superset with
sissy squat   P. 156
3 to 5 supersets
of 10 to 6 repetitions

Calves:
standing   P. 178
calf raise
3 to 5 sets
of 15 to 20 repetitions

Complete Split for Serious Athletes:
Five Days per Week

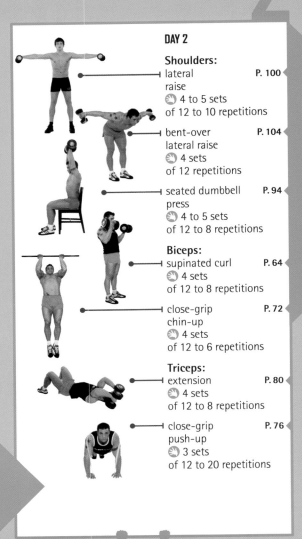

DAY 1

Chest:
bench press   P. 116
4 sets
of 12 to 6 repetitions

crossover   P. 122
with a band
3 sets
of 12 repetitions

push-up   P. 113
3 to 4 sets
of 12 to 6 repetitions

Back:
bent-legged   P. 143
deadlift
4 to 6 sets
of 12 to 6 repetitions

chin-up with bar   P. 131
in front of head
5 sets
of 12 to 6 repetitions

row   P. 134
3 sets
of 12 to 8 repetitions

Forearms:
reverse curl   P. 68
3 to 4 sets
of 20 to 12 repetitions

Abdominals:
twisting crunch   P. 207
4 to 5 sets
of 20 to 25 repetitions

DAY 2

Shoulders:
lateral   P. 100
raise
4 to 5 sets
of 12 to 10 repetitions

bent-over   P. 104
lateral raise
4 sets
of 12 repetitions

seated dumbbell   P. 94
press
4 to 5 sets
of 12 to 8 repetitions

Biceps:
supinated curl   P. 64
4 sets
of 12 to 8 repetitions

close-grip   P. 72
chin-up
4 sets
of 12 to 6 repetitions

Triceps:
extension   P. 80
4 sets
of 12 to 8 repetitions

close-grip   P. 76
push-up
3 sets
of 12 to 20 repetitions

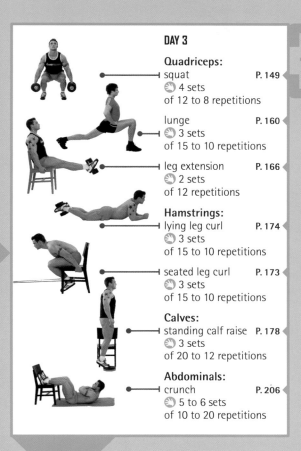

DAY 3

Quadriceps:

squat   P. 149
⟳ 4 sets
of 12 to 8 repetitions

lunge   P. 160
⟳ 3 sets
of 15 to 10 repetitions

leg extension   P. 166
⟳ 2 sets
of 12 repetitions

Hamstrings:

lying leg curl   P. 174
⟳ 3 sets
of 15 to 10 repetitions

seated leg curl   P. 173
⟳ 3 sets
of 15 to 10 repetitions

Calves:

standing calf raise   P. 178
⟳ 3 sets
of 20 to 12 repetitions

Abdominals:

crunch   P. 206
⟳ 5 to 6 sets
of 10 to 20 repetitions

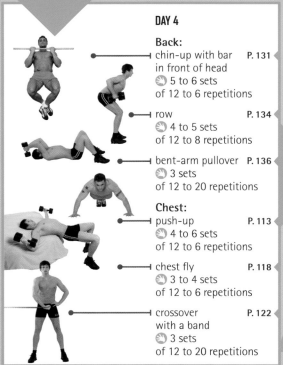

DAY 4

Back:

chin-up with bar   P. 131
in front of head
⟳ 5 to 6 sets
of 12 to 6 repetitions

row   P. 134
⟳ 4 to 5 sets
of 12 to 8 repetitions

bent-arm pullover   P. 136
⟳ 3 sets
of 12 to 20 repetitions

Chest:

push-up   P. 113
⟳ 4 to 6 sets
of 12 to 6 repetitions

chest fly   P. 118
⟳ 3 to 4 sets
of 12 to 6 repetitions

crossover   P. 122
with a band
⟳ 3 sets
of 12 to 20 repetitions

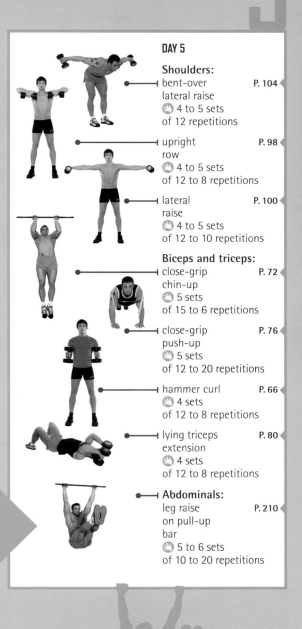

DAY 5

Shoulders:

bent-over   P. 104
lateral raise
⟳ 4 to 5 sets
of 12 repetitions

upright   P. 98
row
⟳ 4 to 5 sets
of 12 to 8 repetitions

lateral   P. 100
raise
⟳ 4 to 5 sets
of 12 to 10 repetitions

Biceps and triceps:

close-grip   P. 72
chin-up
⟳ 5 sets
of 15 to 6 repetitions

close-grip   P. 76
push-up
⟳ 5 sets
of 12 to 20 repetitions

hammer curl   P. 66
⟳ 4 sets
of 12 to 8 repetitions

lying triceps   P. 80
extension
⟳ 4 sets
of 12 to 8 repetitions

Abdominals:

leg raise   P. 210
on pull-up
bar
⟳ 5 to 6 sets
of 10 to 20 repetitions

Specialized Program for the Arms

For anyone who wants to work only on their arms, here is a customized **two-day** program.

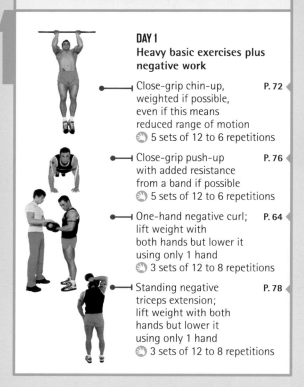

DAY 1
Heavy basic exercises plus negative work

Close-grip chin-up,   P. 72
weighted if possible,
even if this means
reduced range of motion
5 sets of 12 to 6 repetitions

Close-grip push-up   P. 76
with added resistance
from a band if possible
5 sets of 12 to 6 repetitions

One-hand negative curl;   P. 64
lift weight with
both hands but lower it
using only 1 hand
3 sets of 12 to 8 repetitions

Standing negative   P. 78
triceps extension;
lift weight with both
hands but lower it
using only 1 hand
3 sets of 12 to 8 repetitions

DAY 2
Supersets of congestion with strict isolation exercises

Supinated curl   P. 64
in superset
with lying triceps   P. 80
extension
4 supersets
of 20 to 12 repetitions

Hammer curl   P. 66
in superset with
triceps kickback   P. 82
4 supersets
of 20 to 15 repetitions

Reverse curl   P. 68
in superset with
push-down   P. 86
with a band
3 supersets
of 25 to 20 repetitions

20-Minute Athletic Circuit for the Entire Body

Do the exercises as quickly as possible with a minimum amount of rest between sets. You should easily be able to do 3 circuits in less than 20 minutes. When you have gained strength and increased your endurance, you will be able to increase the number of circuits you do during a workout. Do at least **2 workouts per week**.

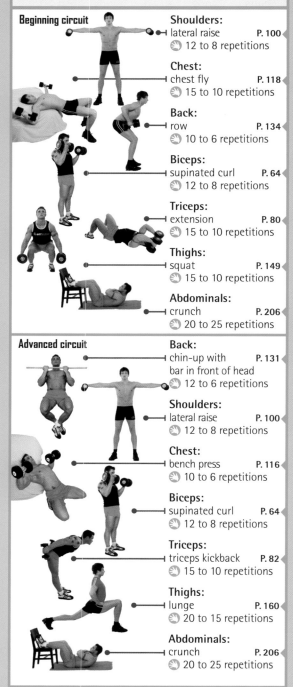

Beginning circuit

Shoulders:
lateral raise   P. 100
12 to 8 repetitions

Chest:
chest fly   P. 118
15 to 10 repetitions

Back:
row   P. 134
10 to 6 repetitions

Biceps:
supinated curl   P. 64
12 to 8 repetitions

Triceps:
extension   P. 80
15 to 10 repetitions

Thighs:
squat   P. 149
15 to 10 repetitions

Abdominals:
crunch   P. 206
20 to 25 repetitions

Advanced circuit

Back:
chin-up with   P. 131
bar in front of head
12 to 6 repetitions

Shoulders:
lateral raise   P. 100
12 to 8 repetitions

Chest:
bench press   P. 116
10 to 6 repetitions

Biceps:
supinated curl   P. 64
12 to 8 repetitions

Triceps:
triceps kickback   P. 82
15 to 10 repetitions

Thighs:
lunge   P. 160
20 to 15 repetitions

Abdominals:
crunch   P. 206
20 to 25 repetitions

Specialized Workout for the Abdominal Muscles

This program is for chiseling the abdominal muscles, losing belly fat, and slimming down the waist. The best way to do this workout is in the morning and the evening so that blood will be circulating in the abdominal muscles throughout the day. Do 2 to 4 circuits per workout without any rest breaks. Your repetitions will be a little quicker than normal, but you should still avoid any jerky movements, particularly in the lower back. You should do 15 to 50 repetitions per set depending on your level of fitness.

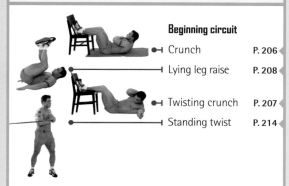

Beginning circuit

Crunch	P. 206
Lying leg raise	P. 208
Twisting crunch	P. 207
Standing twist	P. 214

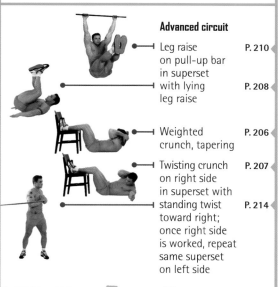

Advanced circuit

Leg raise on pull-up bar in superset with lying leg raise	P. 210 / P. 208
Weighted crunch, tapering	P. 206
Twisting crunch on right side in superset with standing twist toward right; once right side is worked, repeat same superset on left side	P. 207 / P. 214

Women's Strength

Do the following programs for toning muscles in circuits, taking as few rest breaks as possible between the exercises. Beginners can take small rest breaks. After a few workouts, your endurance will improve and these breaks will no longer be necessary.

The advantage of an intense circuit is that it burns the maximum amount of calories in the least amount of time. At the same time, it also helps you maintain excellent physical health, especially cardiovascular health. The goal of each workout is to do the most repetitions possible while reducing the amount of time necessary to do each circuit.

The number of repetitions for each exercise can vary from 25 to 50 depending on your fitness level. It is important to try to reach burn, a sign that your muscles are working deeply and burning the maximum amount of calories. If you are a beginner, your goal is to get as close as possible to 25 repetitions. Even if you do not reach that goal, do not worry. You will make fast progress as you continue to work out. When you can easily do 50 repetitions, you will need to increase the resistance if you want the program to remain effective. Doing 50 repetitions is also a sign that it might be time to move from the beginner program to the advanced program.

Do at least two circuits per workout. Increase the number of circuits as you progress. The total workout time should not exceed 30 minutes. You should do at least two workouts per week, and ideally, you could do four workouts per week. For those who want faster results, daily training is better. In fact, contrary to what you hear or read, there is no miracle program that will give you exceptional results with little effort. Your results will correspond exactly to the amount of time and effort you invest.

You can combine several circuits, for example, glutes circuit plus flat-belly circuit. In this case, you have three choices:

1. Finish the glutes workout before moving on to the abdominal muscles.
2. Alternate circuits by doing a complete circuit for the glutes followed by a complete circuit for the abdomen. Then come back to the glutes circuit. This strategy has the advantage of letting your muscles rest better while you maintain the pace of continuous effort.
3. Work your glutes one day and your waist another day. The only condition is that you do at least two glutes workouts and two abdominal workouts each week to obtain good results.

Program for Firming Up the Glutes

Even though these programs are primarily intended for women, men who want to firm up the buttocks can also use them.

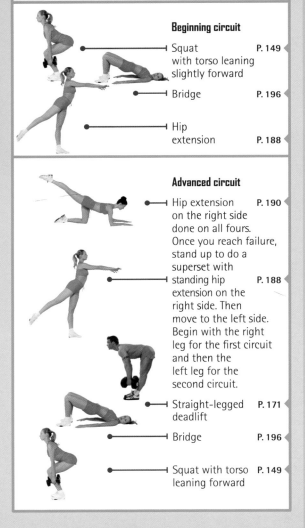

Beginning circuit

Squat with torso leaning slightly forward	P. 149
Bridge	P. 196
Hip extension	P. 188

Advanced circuit

Hip extension P. 190 on the right side done on all fours. Once you reach failure, stand up to do a superset with standing hip P. 188 extension on the right side. Then move to the left side. Begin with the right leg for the first circuit and then the left leg for the second circuit.

Straight-legged deadlift	P. 171
Bridge	P. 196
Squat with torso leaning forward	P. 149

Program for Firming Up the Lower Body

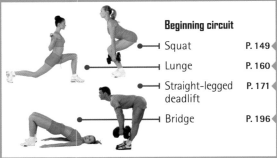

Beginning circuit

Squat	P. 149
Lunge	P. 160
Straight-legged deadlift	P. 171
Bridge	P. 196

Advanced circuit

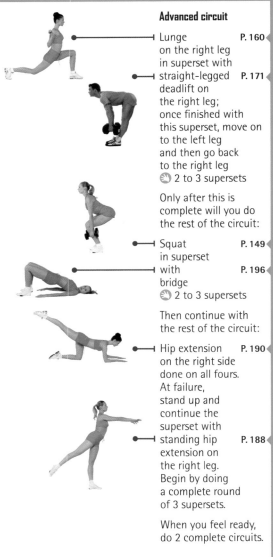

Lunge P. 160 on the right leg in superset with straight-legged P. 171 deadlift on the right leg; once finished with this superset, move on to the left leg and then go back to the right leg 2 to 3 supersets

Only after this is complete will you do the rest of the circuit:

Squat P. 149 in superset with P. 196 bridge 2 to 3 supersets

Then continue with the rest of the circuit:

Hip extension P. 190 on the right side done on all fours. At failure, stand up and continue the superset with standing hip P. 188 extension on the right leg. Begin by doing a complete round of 3 supersets.

When you feel ready, do 2 complete circuits.

Program for a Flat Abdomen

Beginning circuit

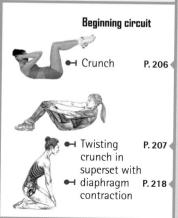

- Crunch P. 206
- Twisting crunch in superset with diaphragm contraction P. 207 / P. 218

Advanced circuit

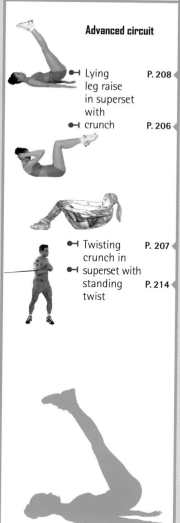

- Lying leg raise in superset with crunch P. 208 / P. 206
- Twisting crunch in superset with standing twist P. 207 / P. 214

Total-Body Firming Program

This program highlights the trouble spots, including the lower body and the abdomen, as well as a few spots on the upper body that are often neglected. For example, large amounts of fat are stored in women's triceps, so these muscles require specific work. The lower-trapezius muscles and the latissimus dorsi muscles are essential parts of the silhouette because they keep the torso from hunching over from the weight of the chest. Therefore, this is an area that should be strengthened.

Do at least 2 circuits twice a week. Ideally, you should be able to do this double circuit in less than 15 minutes. When you feel ready, begin doing 3 and then 4 circuits per workout. When you can do 4 circuits without too much trouble, move on to the advanced program.

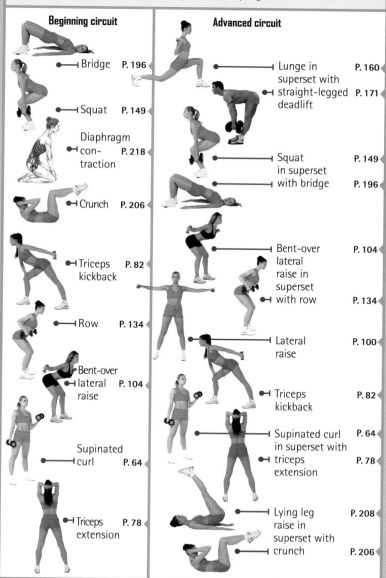

Beginning circuit

- Bridge P. 196
- Squat P. 149
- Diaphragm contraction P. 218
- Crunch P. 206
- Triceps kickback P. 82
- Row P. 134
- Bent-over lateral raise P. 104
- Supinated curl P. 64
- Triceps extension P. 78

Advanced circuit

- Lunge in superset with straight-legged deadlift P. 160 / P. 171
- Squat in superset with bridge P. 149 / P. 196
- Bent-over lateral raise in superset with row P. 104 / P. 134
- Lateral raise P. 100
- Triceps kickback P. 82
- Supinated curl in superset with triceps extension P. 64 / P. 78
- Lying leg raise in superset with crunch P. 208 / P. 206

235

3 Sport-Specific Training

Five Phases of a Training Program

Phase 1: Basic Muscle Conditioning Programs

As a beginner, if you want to improve your physical condition through weight training for one or more sports, here are some basic physical preparation programs. Depending on the program, muscle conditioning focuses on these areas:

> Primarily the thighs
> All the muscles in the body

The main objective of the phase 1 programs is to familiarize yourself with weight training.

Phase 2: Circuit Training

After several weeks of training in phase 1, turn to programs in phase 2 that work the muscles specific to your particular sport. Circuit training begins.

Phase 3: Increasing Volume

After one or two months of adapting to circuit training, it will be time to increase the volume of work. More complex exercises like clean and jerk lifts are introduced into your workouts. The greater number of sets will push you toward splitting your workouts in some cases. This important step corresponds to the programs in phase 3.

Phase 4: More Specialized Training

After three to six months of regular training, you can start to specialize in working the muscles involved in your specific sport. These are the programs in phase 4; there are programs available for a few dozen sports.

Phase 5: Customizing Your Program

After 12 to 18 months of weight training, it is time for you to establish your own training plan as a function of your objectives, your weaknesses, and your priorities. We explain how to proceed when moving into phase 5.

Training in a Circuit or in Sets?

This is a question that you must answer: Is it better to train in a circuit or to train using classic repetitive sets? Scientific studies provide interesting analytical elements. Imagine two groups of beginning tennis players:

1. The first group works on the forehand repetitively. Once they master it, they learn the backhand in the same fashion. This is an example of training in sets.
2. The second group alternates randomly between the forehand and backhand. This is an example of circuit training.

The quantity of forehand and backhand shots done by the two groups at the end of the lesson was identical. Tests for retention were done just after the lesson and then 10 days later. Immediately after the lesson, the players who learned the movements in repetitive sets made the most progress. But 10 days later, the players who trained in a random circuit had improved their game the most.

These results show two things:

1 When you need to learn a new movement quickly, it is better to repeat it in sets. Beginning weight trainers should therefore avoid circuits during the first few weeks of training so that they can learn to perform the exercise. A circuit will only complicate the acquisition of a movement that is already difficult.

2 But if your objective is functional muscles, it quickly becomes better to train in a circuit.

In fact, on the field, it is rare to have to repeat a single movement with the same muscle throughout the whole game. For example, in soccer, even if you primarily use your legs, you have to run forward, backward, and to the sides. You have to dribble and pass the ball. In this case, practicing in a circuit is more suitable than practicing in sets. For a soccer player, we have the following training, consisting of 2 to 5 circuits of 20 to 50 repetitions per exercise:

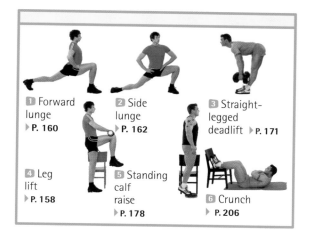

1 Forward lunge
▶ **P. 160**

2 Side lunge
▶ **P. 162**

3 Straight-legged deadlift ▶ **P. 171**

4 Leg lift
▶ **P. 158**

5 Standing calf raise
▶ **P. 178**

6 Crunch
▶ **P. 206**

In other sports, you must simultaneously use your legs and your upper body. This is the case in tennis, rugby, rowing, and swimming. It is simple to develop more sophisticated circuits to meet the difficulty in recruiting the muscles in your upper and lower body. Here is an example of such a circuit that is good for activities requiring total-body work. Do 3 to 6 circuits of 8 to 25 repetitions per exercise:

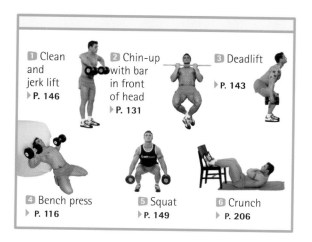

1 Clean and jerk lift
▶ **P. 146**

2 Chin-up with bar in front of head
▶ **P. 131**

3 Deadlift
▶ **P. 143**

4 Bench press
▶ **P. 116**

5 Squat
▶ **P. 149**

6 Crunch
▶ **P. 206**

PHENOMENON OF TRANSFER

Through weight training to improve performance, there will be a transfer between the strength gains achieved in the gym and your athletic prowess on the field or court. For a beginner, this transfer happens pretty well. But the higher the level you are at in your sport, the more this transfer will be problematic.

To ensure an optimal transfer, weight training should be as close as possible to the work required in your sport. This is why it is essential that you adapt your weight training program to your own needs.

Conclusion

When your goal is to put on muscle for aesthetic reasons, it would be counterproductive to do circuit training. Circuit training requires adaptations of the cerebral and nervous systems that are not helpful if you only want to gain muscle mass. In that case, the only reasons to do circuit training would be to save time and to work on increasing endurance and resistance at the same time as muscle mass.

To obtain a functional muscle, the complexity of your weight training routine must approach the complexity encountered on the field. In this way your training will prepare not only your muscles but also your nervous system for the technical difficulties you will encounter in your sport.

Phase 1: Basic Muscle Conditioning Programs

You should follow the phase 1 program for several weeks so that you can learn to master the most common weight training movements. When you feel comfortable, you can move on to circuit training (phase 2).

Basic Program for Sports That Primarily Require the Thighs
(Soccer, Running, Biking, and Downhill Skiing)
2 or 3 workouts per week

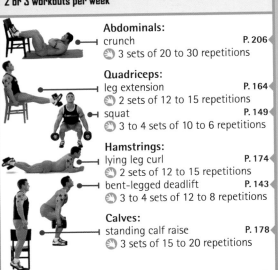

Abdominals:
crunch   P. 206
3 sets of 20 to 30 repetitions

Quadriceps:
leg extension   P. 164
2 sets of 12 to 15 repetitions
squat   P. 149
3 to 4 sets of 10 to 6 repetitions

Hamstrings:
lying leg curl   P. 174
2 sets of 12 to 15 repetitions
bent-legged deadlift   P. 143
3 to 4 sets of 12 to 8 repetitions

Calves:
standing calf raise   P. 178
3 sets of 15 to 20 repetitions

Basic Program for Sports That Require the Thighs Plus Upper-Body Muscles
(Rugby, Rowing, Racquetball, Combat Sports, and Cross-Country Skiing)
2 or 3 workouts per week

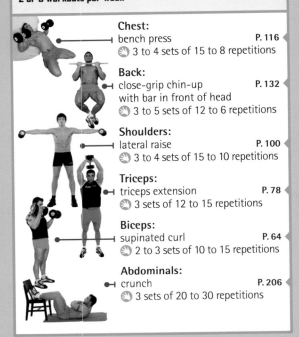

Chest:
bench press   P. 116
3 to 4 sets of 15 to 8 repetitions

Back:
close-grip chin-up
with bar in front of head   P. 132
3 to 5 sets of 12 to 6 repetitions

Shoulders:
lateral raise   P. 100
3 to 4 sets of 15 to 10 repetitions

Triceps:
triceps extension   P. 78
3 sets of 12 to 15 repetitions

Biceps:
supinated curl   P. 64
2 to 3 sets of 10 to 15 repetitions

Abdominals:
crunch   P. 206
3 sets of 20 to 30 repetitions

Phase 2: Circuit Training

After doing the phase 1 program for one to two months, it is time to move toward circuit training.

Basic Circuit for Sports That Primarily Require the Thighs
Do 2 to 5 circuits of the following:
- 10 to 20 repetitions in sports requiring strength
- 25 to 50 repetitions in sports requiring considerable endurance
Repeat this workout 2 or 3 times per week.

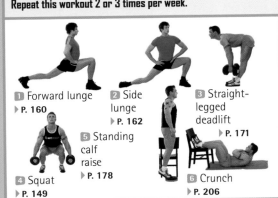

1 Forward lunge
▶ P. 160

2 Side lunge
▶ P. 162

3 Straight-legged deadlift
▶ P. 171

5 Standing calf raise
▶ P. 178

4 Squat
▶ P. 149

6 Crunch
▶ P. 206

Basic Circuit for Sports That Require the Thighs Plus Upper-Body Muscles
Do 3 to 5 circuits of the following:
- 15 to 25 repetitions in sports requiring strength
- 25 to 50 repetitions in sports requiring endurance
Repeat this workout 2 to 3 times per week.

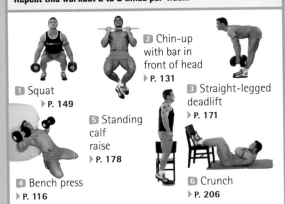

1 Squat
▶ P. 149

2 Chin-up with bar in front of head
▶ P. 131

3 Straight-legged deadlift
▶ P. 171

5 Standing calf raise
▶ P. 178

4 Bench press
▶ P. 116

6 Crunch
▶ P. 206

Phase 3: Increasing Volume

After about three to six months of basic circuit training, you can increase the volume of work so that you continue to progress. It is also time to introduce more complex exercises that require better control, such as clean and jerk lifts.

Advanced Circuit for Sports That Primarily Require the Thighs

🔄 Do 3 to 6 circuits of the following:
- 10 to 20 repetitions in sports requiring strength
- 25 to 50 repetitions in sports requiring endurance

Ideally, you should ensure that you constantly rotate and alternate exercises so that you increase the difficulty of your workout. Do workout A one or two times per week. Alternate it with workout B for a program that resembles this:

Note: A crossed-out box indicates a rest day.

Day	☀	1	2	3	4	5	6	7
Workout	🔗	A	✕	B	✕	A/B	✕	✕

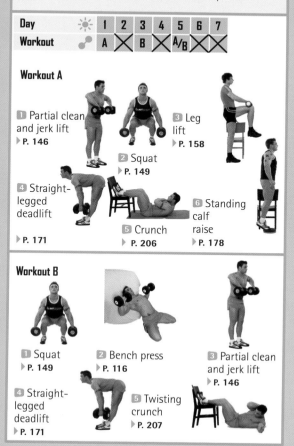

Workout A

1 Partial clean and jerk lift
▶ P. 146

2 Squat
▶ P. 149

3 Leg lift
▶ P. 158

4 Straight-legged deadlift
▶ P. 171

5 Crunch
▶ P. 206

6 Standing calf raise
▶ P. 178

Workout B

1 Squat
▶ P. 149

2 Bench press
▶ P. 116

3 Partial clean and jerk lift
▶ P. 146

4 Straight-legged deadlift
▶ P. 171

5 Twisting crunch
▶ P. 207

Advanced Circuit for Sports That Require the Thighs Plus Upper-Body Muscles

🔄 Do 4 to 6 circuits of the following:
- 10 to 20 repetitions in sports requiring strength
- 25 to 50 repetitions in sports requiring endurance

Ensure that you rotate between the four workouts throughout the weeks. You can begin to personalize the workouts on days 5 and 12, because the choice of workout A or B will depend on the muscles (upper or lower body) that are most important in your sport. After two weeks, start the cycle over again.

☀	1	2	3	4	5	6	7	8	9	10	11	12	13	14
🔗	A¹	✕	B¹	✕	A²/B²	✕	✕	A²	✕	B²	✕	A¹/B¹	✕	✕

A Workouts (focus on upper-body muscles)
Workout A¹

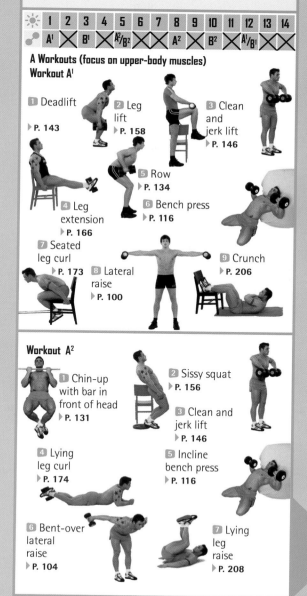

1 Deadlift
▶ P. 143

2 Leg lift
▶ P. 158

3 Clean and jerk lift
▶ P. 146

4 Leg extension
▶ P. 166

5 Row
▶ P. 134

6 Bench press
▶ P. 116

7 Seated leg curl
▶ P. 173

8 Lateral raise
▶ P. 100

9 Crunch
▶ P. 206

Workout A²

1 Chin-up with bar in front of head
▶ P. 131

2 Sissy squat
▶ P. 156

3 Clean and jerk lift
▶ P. 146

4 Lying leg curl
▶ P. 174

5 Incline bench press
▶ P. 116

6 Bent-over lateral raise
▶ P. 104

7 Lying leg raise
▶ P. 208

Advanced Circuit for Sports That Require the Thighs Plus Upper-Body Muscles

B Workouts (focus on lower-body muscles)
Workout B¹

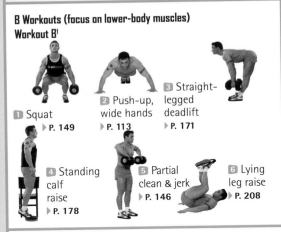

1 Squat ▶ P. 149
2 Push-up, wide hands ▶ P. 113
3 Straight-legged deadlift ▶ P. 171
4 Standing calf raise ▶ P. 178
5 Partial clean & jerk ▶ P. 146
6 Lying leg raise ▶ P. 208

Workout B²

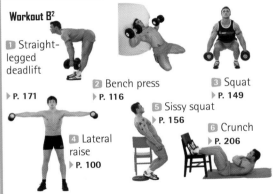

1 Straight-legged deadlift ▶ P. 171
2 Bench press ▶ P. 116
3 Squat ▶ P. 149
4 Lateral raise ▶ P. 100
5 Sissy squat ▶ P. 156
6 Crunch ▶ P. 206

IMPORTANCE OF TORSO ROTATION FOR PERFORMANCE

There are many sports in which movement is initiated by the rotation of the torso. For example, the power of a golfer's swing is acquired during the windup when he brings his club as high as possible before lowering it to hit the ball. For a boxer, the punch is initiated by a rotation of the torso to the back as a kind of windup. So it is important to exercise the muscles responsible for this rotation so that you can do the following:

> Gain power
> Strengthen the muscles to prevent injuries that are very common in this relatively fragile area

Beginning Program for Strengthening the Rotator Muscles in the Torso
Do 2 to 4 circuits of 25 to 50 repetitions.

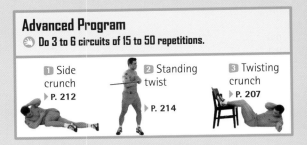

1 Standing twist ▶ P. 214
2 Twisting crunch ▶ P. 207

Advanced Program
Do 3 to 6 circuits of 15 to 50 repetitions.

1 Side crunch ▶ P. 212
2 Standing twist ▶ P. 214
3 Twisting crunch ▶ P. 207

Phase 4: More Specialized Training

After six to eight months of regular training, it is time to focus more specifically on the muscles involved in your particular sport. In fact, every sport requires the use of different muscles. You should also be able to modify the sample programs and substitute some exercises for ones that are most beneficial to you.

Plyometric exercises are also introduced at the beginning of training to sharpen the nervous system response and facilitate explosiveness in your muscles. Do these exercises after a good total-body warm-up. Remember that the rule for plyometrics is to do the maximum number of repetitions until you lose the explosiveness in your muscles. Then you must stop the set and rest for 30 to 60 seconds before moving to the next set.

After working out, you should do some stretching exercises. Hold the stretch for 10 to 60 seconds before moving to the next stretch. In general, you should do 1 to 3 sets of a stretching exercise per muscle group unless it is specified that a muscle needs to be stretched from several angles.

So that you can find the program best suited for you, we have included 16 broad disciplines that cover the majority of the most common sports. You can certainly rotate exercises from workout to workout to increase the level of difficulty.

Soccer

The goal of this program is to strengthen the thighs as well as protect the lumbar region, knees, and hip rotator muscles.

🔄 **Do 2 to 5 circuits of 20 to 50 repetitions.**

• **Do each workout 1 or 2 times per week, preferably repeating workout A.**

Workout A

Preworkout plyometric exercises
▶ **P. 167**
🔄 3 or 4 sets with maximum repetitions per exercise

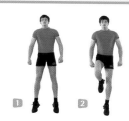

1 Box squat with pause at bottom, tapering
▶ **P. 150**

2 Crunch
▶ **P. 206**

3 Straight-legged deadlift, tapering
▶ **P. 171**

4 Seated inner-thigh rotation using continuous tension
▶ **P. 201**

5 Seated outer-thigh rotation using continuous tension
▶ **P. 201**

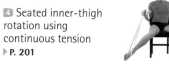

6 Seated thigh adduction using continuous tension
▶ **P. 165**

7 Leg lift using continuous tension
▶ **P. 158**

Postworkout stretches
▶ **PP. 137/162/165/185/176**

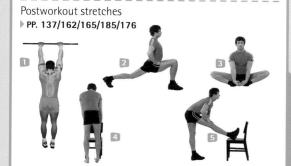

Workout B

Preworkout plyometric exercises
▶ **P. 167**
🔄 3 or 4 sets with maximum repetitions per exercise

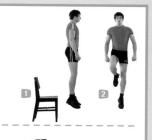

1 Partial clean and jerk lift
▶ **P. 146**

2 Lying leg raise
▶ **P. 208**

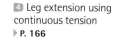

3 Bent-over lateral raise
▶ **P. 104**

4 Leg extension using continuous tension
▶ **P. 166**

5 Crunch
▶ **P. 206**

6 Seated leg curl using continuous tension
▶ **P. 173**

7 Twisting crunch
▶ **P. 207**

8 Standing calf raise using continuous tension
▶ **P. 178**

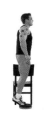

Postworkout stretches
▶ **PP. 106/137/178/176/201**

241

Cycling

The goal of this program is to strengthen the thighs and protect the back.

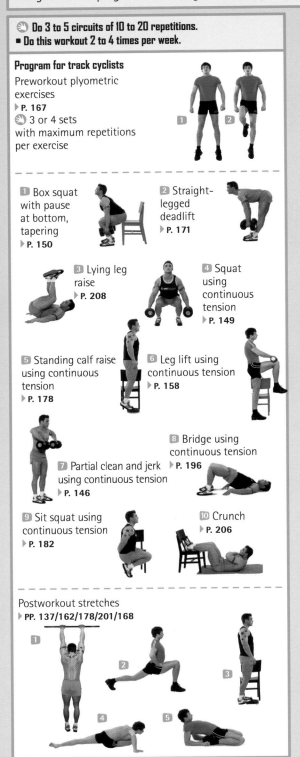

🌀 **Do 3 to 5 circuits of 10 to 20 repetitions.**
■ **Do this workout 2 to 4 times per week.**

Program for track cyclists

Preworkout plyometric exercises
▶ **P. 167**
🌀 3 or 4 sets with maximum repetitions per exercise

1 2

1 **Box squat with pause at bottom, tapering**
▶ **P. 150**

2 **Straight-legged deadlift**
▶ **P. 171**

3 **Lying leg raise**
▶ **P. 208**

4 **Squat using continuous tension**
▶ **P. 149**

5 **Standing calf raise using continuous tension**
▶ **P. 178**

6 **Leg lift using continuous tension**
▶ **P. 158**

7 **Partial clean and jerk using continuous tension**
▶ **P. 146**

8 **Bridge using continuous tension**
▶ **P. 196**

9 **Sit squat using continuous tension**
▶ **P. 182**

10 **Crunch**
▶ **P. 206**

Postworkout stretches
▶ **PP. 137/162/178/201/168**

1 2 3 4 5

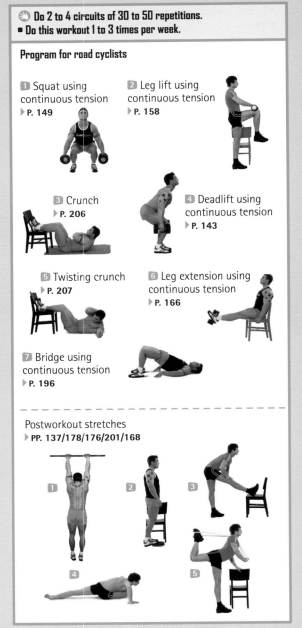

🌀 **Do 2 to 4 circuits of 30 to 50 repetitions.**
■ **Do this workout 1 to 3 times per week.**

Program for road cyclists

1 **Squat using continuous tension**
▶ **P. 149**

2 **Leg lift using continuous tension**
▶ **P. 158**

3 **Crunch**
▶ **P. 206**

4 **Deadlift using continuous tension**
▶ **P. 143**

5 **Twisting crunch**
▶ **P. 207**

6 **Leg extension using continuous tension**
▶ **P. 166**

7 **Bridge using continuous tension**
▶ **P. 196**

Postworkout stretches
▶ **PP. 137/178/176/201/168**

1 2 3 4 5

Racket Sports

The goal of this program is to strengthen the thighs and arms while protecting the shoulders and hamstrings.
- **Do each workout 1 or 2 times per week with a preference for workout A.**

Workout A

Preworkout plyometric exercises
▶ **PP. 167/124**
🔄 3 or 4 sets with maximum repetitions per exercise

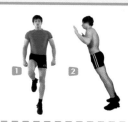

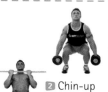

1 Semisquat using continuous tension
▶ **P. 149**

2 Chin-up with bar in front of head
▶ **P. 131**

3 Complete clean and jerk lift using continuous tension
▶ **P. 146**

4 Shoulder rotation with a band using continuous tension
▶ **P. 111**

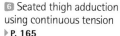

5 Seated inner-thigh rotation using continuous tension
▶ **P. 201**

6 Seated thigh adduction using continuous tension
▶ **P. 165**

7 Crunch
▶ **P. 206**

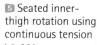

8 Standing calf raise using continuous tension
▶ **P. 178**

Postworkout stretches
▶ **PP. 106/137/91/87/185/162**

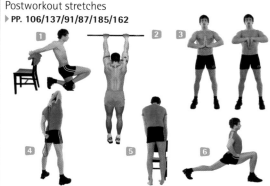

Workout B

Preworkout plyometric exercises
▶ **PP. 167/124**
🔄 3 or 4 sets with maximum repetitions per exercise

1 Straight-legged deadlift
▶ **P. 171**

2 Standing twist
▶ **P. 214**

3 Row
▶ **P. 134**

4 Side crunch
▶ **P. 212**

5 Bent-over lateral raise
▶ **P. 104**

6 Twisting crunch
▶ **P. 207**

7 Seated leg curl using continuous tension
▶ **P. 173**

8 Leg lift using continuous tension
▶ **P. 158**

Postworkout stretches
▶ **PP. 106/137/91/87/165/176**

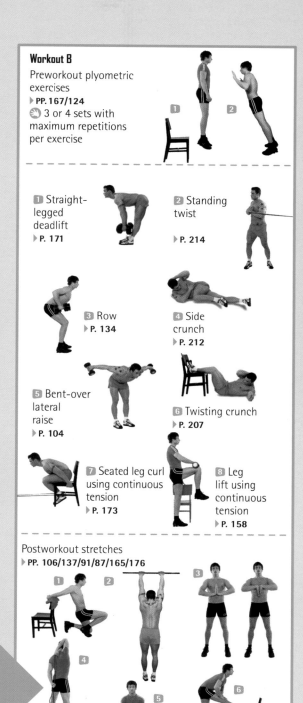

Football and Rugby

The goal of this program is to strengthen the thighs, torso muscles, and arms while protecting the neck, back, knees, and hamstrings.

🏃 Do 2 to 5 circuits of 10 to 30 repetitions.
● Do each workout 1 or 2 times per week with a preference for repeating workout A.

Workout A

Preworkout plyometric exercises
▶ PP. 167/124
🏃 3 or 4 sets with maximum repetitions per exercise

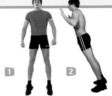

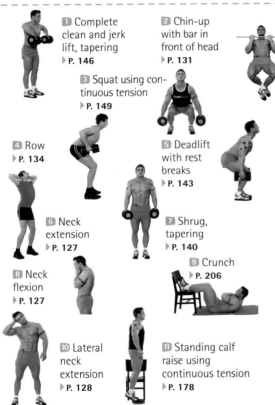

1 Complete clean and jerk lift, tapering
▶ P. 146

2 Chin-up with bar in front of head
▶ P. 131

3 Squat using continuous tension
▶ P. 149

4 Row
▶ P. 134

5 Deadlift with rest breaks
▶ P. 143

6 Neck extension
▶ P. 127

7 Shrug, tapering
▶ P. 140

8 Neck flexion
▶ P. 127

9 Crunch
▶ P. 206

10 Lateral neck extension
▶ P. 128

11 Standing calf raise using continuous tension
▶ P. 178

Postworkout stretches
▶ PP. 176/162/106/185/137

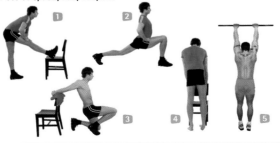

Workout B

Preworkout plyometric exercises
▶ PP. 167/124
🏃 3 or 4 sets with maximum repetitions per exercise

1 Box squat with pause at bottom
▶ P. 150

2 Standing twist
▶ P. 214

3 Bench press using continuous tension
▶ P. 116

4 Straight-legged deadlift, tapering
▶ P. 171

5 Twisting crunch
▶ P. 207

6 Bent-over lateral raise
▶ P. 104

7 Seated inner-thigh rotation using continuous tension
▶ P. 201

8 Shoulder rotation with a band
▶ P. 111

9 Seated leg curl using continuous tension
▶ P. 173

10 Lying leg raise
▶ P. 208

Postworkout stretches
▶ PP. 176/162/106/185/137

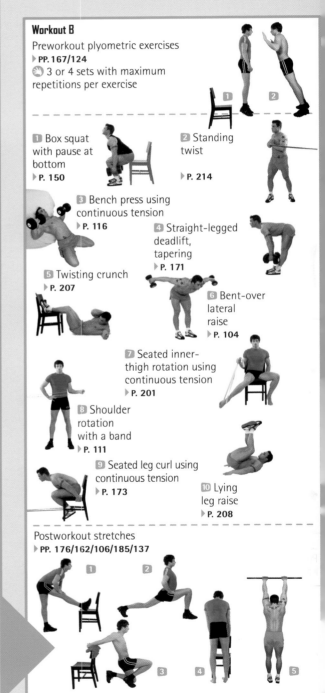

Basketball, Volleyball, and Handball

The goal of this program is to strengthen the thighs, shoulders, and arms while protecting the knees and hamstrings.

👋 **Do 2 to 4 circuits of 20 to 50 repetitions.**
■ **Do this workout 2 or 3 times per week.**

Workout A

Preworkout plyometric exercises
▶ **PP. 167/124**
👋 3 or 4 sets with maximum repetitions per exercise

1 Complete clean and jerk
▶ **P. 146**

2 Chin-up with bar in front of head
▶ **P. 131**

3 Semisquat using continuous tension
▶ **P. 149**

4 Twisting crunch
▶ **P. 207**

5 Straight-legged deadlift, tapering
▶ **P. 171**

6 Standing twist
▶ **P. 214**

7 Bent-over lateral raise
▶ **P. 104**

8 Standing calf raise using continuous tension
▶ **P. 178**

9 Seated inner-thigh rotation
▶ **P. 201**

10 Seated leg curl using continuous tension
▶ **P. 173**

11 Shoulder rotation with a band
▶ **P. 111**

Postworkout stretches
▶ **PP. 137/91/87/162**

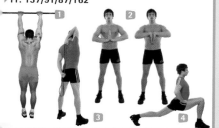

Alpine Sports: Downhill Skiing and Cross-Country Skiing

The goal of this program is to strengthen the thighs and protect the back, knees, and hamstrings.

👋 **Do 2 to 4 circuits of 25 to 40 repetitions for downhill skiing and 30 to 100 repetitions for cross-country skiing.**
■ **Do this workout 2 or 3 times per week.**

Downhill skiing circuit

Preworkout plyometric exercises ▶ **P. 167**
👋 5 or 6 sets with maximum repetitions per exercise

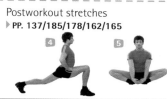

1 Semi-squat with constant tension
▶ **P. 149**

2 Bent-over lateral raise
▶ **P. 104**

3 Deadlift using continuous tension
▶ **P. 143**

4 Seated thigh adduction using continuous tension
▶ **P. 165**

5 Row
▶ **P. 134**

6 Seated leg curl using continuous tension
▶ **P. 173**

7 Lying leg raise
▶ **P. 208**

8 Standing calf raise using continuous tension
▶ **P. 178**

Postworkout stretches
▶ **PP. 137/185/178/162/165**

Cross-country skiing circuit

1 Lunge alternating left and right legs for each repetition
▶ **P. 160**

2 Bent-over lateral raise
▶ **P. 104**

3 Deadlift using continuous tension
▶ **P. 143**

4 Shoulder rotation with a band
▶ **P. 111**

5 Seated thigh adduction using continuous tension
▶ **P. 165**

6 Lying leg raise
▶ **P. 208**

7 Seated leg curl using continuous tension
▶ **P. 173**

8 Standing calf raise using continuous tension
▶ **P. 178**

Postworkout stretches
▶ **PP. 106/162/165/185/137/178**

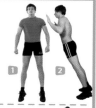
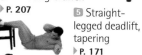
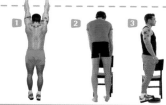
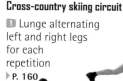
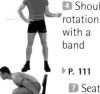
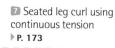

Combat Sports

The goal of this program is to strengthen all the muscles in the body while protecting the main joints.

Gripping combat sports: wrestling, judo, and ultimate fighting

Do each workout 1 or 2 times per week, with a preference for workout A.

Do 3 to 6 circuits of 20 to 40 repetitions.

Workout A

Preworkout plyometric exercises
▶ PP. 167/124/167
2 or 3 sets with maximum repetitions per exercise

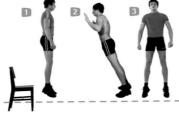

1 Complete clean and jerk with rest breaks
▶ P. 146

2 Standing twist
▶ P. 214

3 Semisquat using continuous tension
▶ P. 149

4 Chin-up with bar in front of head with rest breaks
▶ P. 131

5 Standing calf raise
▶ P. 178

6 Hammer curl
▶ P. 66

7 Twisting crunch
▶ P. 207

8 Standing twist
▶ P. 214

9 Neck extension
▶ P. 127

10 Neck flexion
▶ P. 127

11 Lateral neck extension
▶ P. 128

Postworkout stretches
▶ PP. 106/165/137/12/91

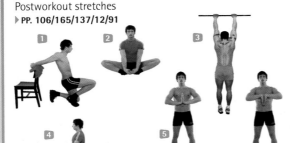

Workout B

Preworkout plyometric exercises
▶ P. 167
4 or 5 sets with maximum repetitions per exercise

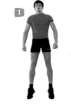

1 Bench press
▶ P. 116

2 Straight-legged deadlift, tapering
▶ P. 171

3 Row
▶ P. 134

4 Lying leg raise
▶ P. 208

5 Supinated curl, tapering
▶ P. 64

6 Wrist curl
▶ P. 88

7 Crunch
▶ P. 206

8 Seated inner-thigh rotation
▶ P. 201

9 Seated outer-thigh rotation
▶ P. 201

10 Seated thigh adduction using continuous tension
▶ P. 165

11 Shrug, changing placement of dumbbells (begin with dumbbells behind back, then at sides, and finish with dumbbells in front)
▶ P. 140

Postworkout stretches
▶ PP. 106/185/137/91/12

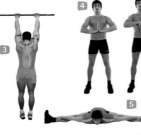

Boxing

Do 2 to 5 circuits of 10 to 50 repetitions. Do this workout 2 or 3 times per week.

Preworkout plyometric exercises
▶ PP. 167/124
5 or 6 sets with maximum repetitions per exercise

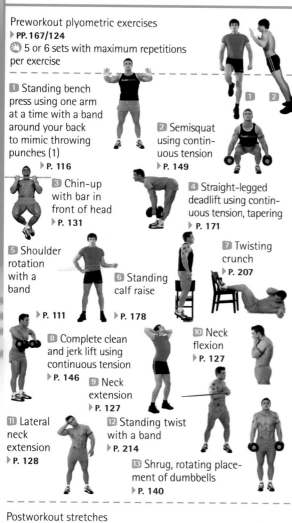

1 Standing bench press using one arm at a time with a band around your back to mimic throwing punches (1)
▶ P. 116

2 Semisquat using continuous tension
▶ P. 149

3 Chin-up with bar in front of head
▶ P. 131

4 Straight-legged deadlift using continuous tension, tapering
▶ P. 171

5 Shoulder rotation with a band
▶ P. 111

6 Standing calf raise
▶ P. 178

7 Twisting crunch
▶ P. 207

8 Complete clean and jerk lift using continuous tension
▶ P. 146

9 Neck extension
▶ P. 127

10 Neck flexion
▶ P. 127

11 Lateral neck extension
▶ P. 128

12 Standing twist with a band
▶ P. 214

13 Shrug, rotating placement of dumbbells
▶ P. 140

Postworkout stretches
▶ PP. 106/162/137/91/185

(1) *Note:* You often see this exercise done while holding dumbbells. Unfortunately, the resistance provided by the weights is applied from top to bottom and not from back to front as it is in boxing. Only the band can provide the explosiveness required for punching.

Track and Field: Sprints, Running, Jumping, and Shot Put

The goal of this program is to strengthen the thighs while protecting the back, hips, hamstrings, and shoulders.

Sprints and foot races

Do 2 to 5 circuits of the following:
- 10 to 20 repetitions for sprinters
- 20 to 40 repetitions for races from 1 to 5 minutes
- 50 to 100 repetitions for longer races

Do this workout 2 or 3 times per week.

Preworkout plyometric exercises
▶ P. 167
5 or 6 sets with maximum repetitions per exercise

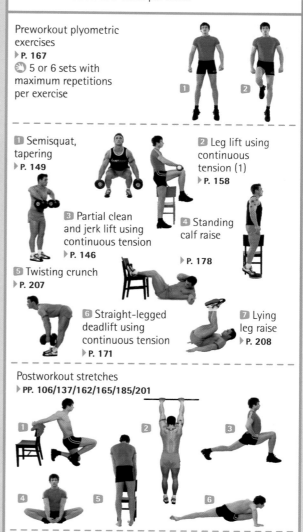

1 Semisquat, tapering
▶ P. 149

2 Leg lift using continuous tension (1)
▶ P. 158

3 Partial clean and jerk lift using continuous tension
▶ P. 146

4 Standing calf raise
▶ P. 178

5 Twisting crunch
▶ P. 207

6 Straight-legged deadlift using continuous tension
▶ P. 171

7 Lying leg raise
▶ P. 208

Postworkout stretches
▶ PP. 106/137/162/165/185/201

(1) *Note:* When doing leg lifts, hold onto the chair as little as possible so that you will be forced to stabilize yourself by contracting your gluteus medius near the thigh of the standing leg. This muscle is very important during a race, and it prevents the pelvis from moving to the opposite side. The tensor fasciae latae will also be stimulated. This muscle lifts the thigh and also sheathes the external part of the quadriceps, which provides strength during a race.

Shot Put

The goal of this program is to strengthen the thighs, rotator muscles in the torso, and shoulders while protecting the back and shoulder joints.

Do 4 to 6 circuits of 1 to 6 repetitions. Do this workout 3 to 5 times per week.

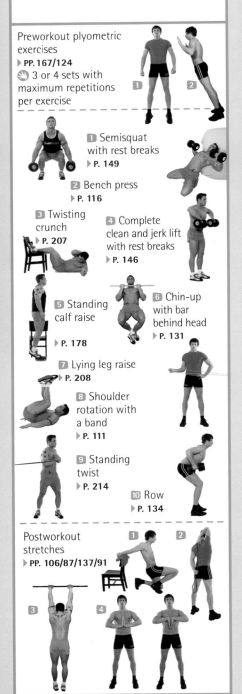

Preworkout plyometric exercises
▶ PP. 167/124
3 or 4 sets with maximum repetitions per exercise

1 Semisquat with rest breaks
▶ P. 149

2 Bench press
▶ P. 116

3 Twisting crunch
▶ P. 207

4 Complete clean and jerk lift with rest breaks
▶ P. 146

5 Standing calf raise
▶ P. 178

6 Chin-up with bar behind head
▶ P. 131

7 Lying leg raise
▶ P. 208

8 Shoulder rotation with a band
▶ P. 111

9 Standing twist
▶ P. 214

10 Row
▶ P. 134

Postworkout stretches
▶ PP. 106/87/137/91

Swimming

The goal of this program is to strengthen the shoulders, chest, back, and thighs while protecting the primary joints.

Do 4 to 6 circuits of 25 to 75 repetitions.
Do this workout 2 to 4 times per week.

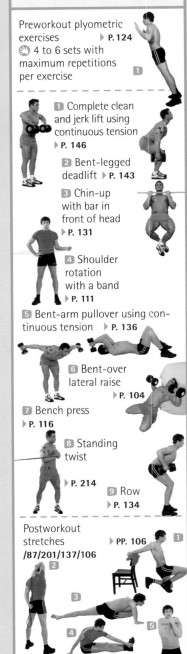

Preworkout plyometric exercises
▶ P. 124
4 to 6 sets with maximum repetitions per exercise

1 Complete clean and jerk lift using continuous tension
▶ P. 146

2 Bent-legged deadlift ▶ P. 143

3 Chin-up with bar in front of head
▶ P. 131

4 Shoulder rotation with a band
▶ P. 111

5 Bent-arm pullover using continuous tension ▶ P. 136

6 Bent-over lateral raise
▶ P. 104

7 Bench press
▶ P. 116

8 Standing twist
▶ P. 214

9 Row
▶ P. 134

Postworkout stretches ▶ PP. 106/87/201/137/106

Golf

The goal of this program is to strengthen the rotator muscles in the torso while protecting the back, shoulders, and hips.

Do 2 to 3 circuits of 10 to 20 repetitions.
Do this workout 1 to 2 times per week.

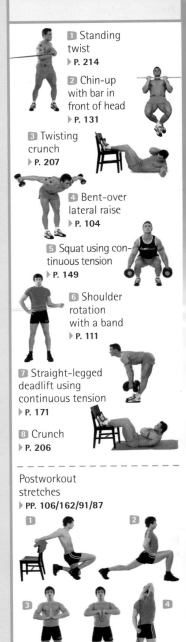

1 Standing twist
▶ P. 214

2 Chin-up with bar in front of head
▶ P. 131

3 Twisting crunch
▶ P. 207

4 Bent-over lateral raise
▶ P. 104

5 Squat using continuous tension
▶ P. 149

6 Shoulder rotation with a band
▶ P. 111

7 Straight-legged deadlift using continuous tension
▶ P. 171

8 Crunch
▶ P. 206

Postworkout stretches
▶ PP. 106/162/91/87

Ice Sports: Ice Skating and Hockey

The goal of this program is to strengthen the thighs, glutes, and rotator muscles of the torso while protecting the lumbar region and the hamstrings.

- Do 2 to 5 circuits of 10 to 40 repetitions.
- Do this workout 2 to 3 times per week.

Solo ice skating

Preworkout plyometric exercises
▶ PP. 167/124
2 or 3 sets with maximum repetitions per exercise

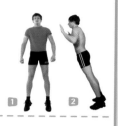

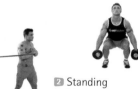

1 Squat using continuous tension
▶ P. 149

2 Standing twist
▶ P. 214

3 Straight-legged deadlift
▶ P. 171

4 Twisting crunch
▶ P. 207

5 Seated inner-thigh rotation
▶ P. 201

6 Seated outer-thigh rotation
▶ P. 201

7 Seated thigh adduction
▶ P. 165

8 Standing calf raise using continuous tension
▶ P. 178

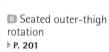

Postworkout stretches
▶ PP. 106/165/137/12/162

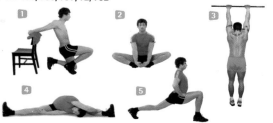
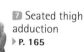

Skating in team sports

Preworkout plyometric exercises
▶ PP. 167/124
3 or 4 sets with maximum repetitions per exercise

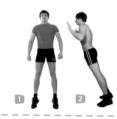

1 Complete clean and jerk using continuous tension
▶ P. 146

2 Semisquat
▶ P. 149

3 Chin-up with bar in front of head
▶ P. 131

4 Standing twist
▶ P. 214

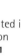
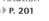

5 Seated inner-thigh rotation
▶ P. 201

6 Twisting crunch
▶ P. 207

7 Seated outer-thigh rotation using continuous tension
▶ P. 201

1

8 Standing calf raise using continuous tension
▶ P. 178

9 Seated thigh adduction
▶ P. 165

Postworkout stretches
▶ PP. 106/137/91/12

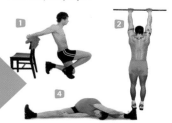
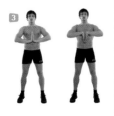

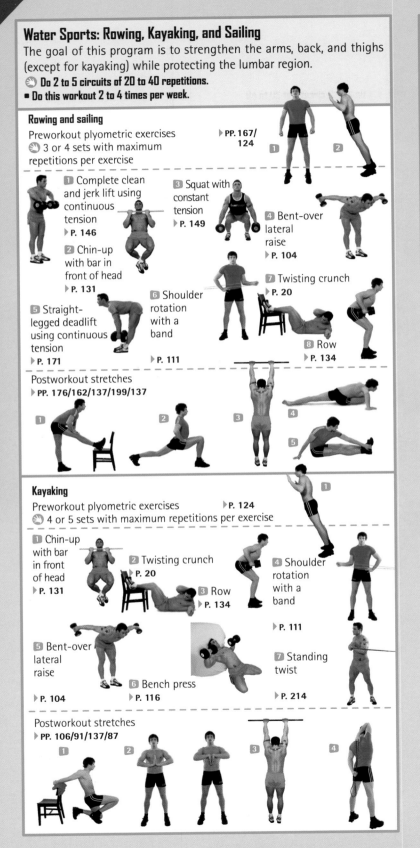
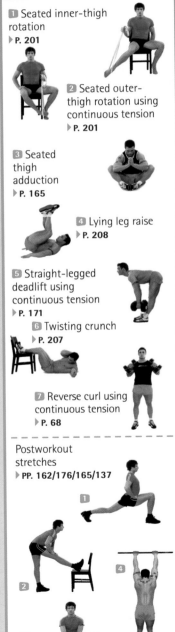

Water Sports: Rowing, Kayaking, and Sailing

The goal of this program is to strengthen the arms, back, and thighs (except for kayaking) while protecting the lumbar region.

- Do 2 to 5 circuits of 20 to 40 repetitions.
- Do this workout 2 to 4 times per week.

Rowing and sailing

Preworkout plyometric exercises ▶ PP. 167/124
- 3 or 4 sets with maximum repetitions per exercise

1 Complete clean and jerk lift using continuous tension ▶ P. 146

2 Chin-up with bar in front of head ▶ P. 131

3 Squat with constant tension ▶ P. 149

4 Bent-over lateral raise ▶ P. 104

5 Straight-legged deadlift using continuous tension ▶ P. 171

6 Shoulder rotation with a band ▶ P. 111

7 Twisting crunch ▶ P. 20

8 Row ▶ P. 134

Postworkout stretches ▶ PP. 176/162/137/199/137

Kayaking

Preworkout plyometric exercises ▶ P. 124
- 4 or 5 sets with maximum repetitions per exercise

1 Chin-up with bar in front of head ▶ P. 131

2 Twisting crunch ▶ P. 20

3 Row ▶ P. 134

4 Shoulder rotation with a band ▶ P. 111

5 Bent-over lateral raise ▶ P. 104

6 Bench press ▶ P. 116

7 Standing twist ▶ P. 214

Postworkout stretches ▶ PP. 106/91/137/87

Horseback Riding

The goal of this program is to protect the back (especially the lumbar region) and the adductor muscles as well as to strengthen the thighs.

- Do 2 or 3 circuits of 20 to 50 repetitions.
- Do this workout 1 or 2 times per week.

1 Seated inner-thigh rotation ▶ P. 201

2 Seated outer-thigh rotation using continuous tension ▶ P. 201

3 Seated thigh adduction ▶ P. 165

4 Lying leg raise ▶ P. 208

5 Straight-legged deadlift using continuous tension ▶ P. 171

6 Twisting crunch ▶ P. 207

7 Reverse curl using continuous tension ▶ P. 68

Postworkout stretches ▶ PP. 162/176/165/137

Arm Wrestling

The goal of this program is to strengthen the arms as well as the rotator muscles in the arms while protecting the shoulders, elbows, and forearms.

🏋 **Do 4 to 6 circuits of 3 to 12 repetitions.**
▪ **Do this workout 2 to 4 times per week.**

Preworkout plyometric exercises
▶ **P. 124**
🏋 2 or 3 sets with maximum repetitions per exercise ❶

❶ Weighted chin-up, using rest breaks
▶ **P. 131**
❷ Bench press, tapering
▶ **P. 116**
❸ Unilateral hammer curl (1), tapering
▶ **P. 66**
❹ Shoulder rotation with a band
▶ **P. 111**
❺ Unilateral row (1), tapering
▶ **P. 134**
❻ Unilateral curl (1), tapering
▶ **P. 64**
❼ Wrist extension using continuous tension
▶ **P. 90**
❽ Unilateral reverse curl (1) using continuous tension
▶ **P. 68**
❾ Wrist curl using continuous tension
▶ **P. 88**
❿ Weighted crunch, tapering
▶ **P. 206**

Postworkout stretches
▶ **PP. 106/87/137/91**

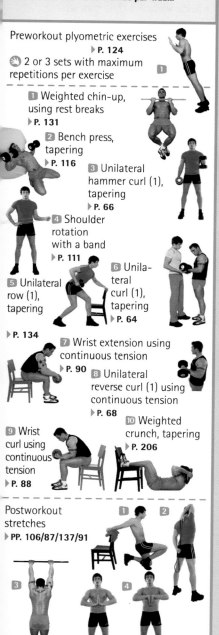

(1) *Note:* with emphasis on the arm you use to compete.

Climbing

The goal of this program is to strengthen the thighs, arms, forearms, and back.

🏋 **Do 2 or 3 circuits of 20 to 40 repetitions.**
▪ **Do this workout 1 or 2 times per week. Use tapering sets extensively for best results.**

❶ Chin-up, tapering
▶ **P. 131**
❷ Squat using continuous tension
▶ **P. 149**
❸ Bench press using continuous tension
▶ **P. 116**
❹ Deadlift
▶ **P. 143**
❺ Shoulder rotation with a band
▶ **P. 111**
❻ Standing calf raise using continuous tension
▶ **P. 178**
❼ Hammer curl, tapering
▶ **P. 66**
❽ Wrist extension, tapering
▶ **P. 90**
❾ Crunch ▶ **P. 206**
❿ Wrist curl, tapering ▶ **P. 88**

Postworkout stretches ▶ **PP. 106/162/137 /91/185**

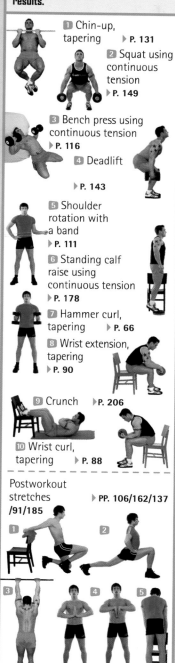

Auto Sports and Motorcycling

The goal of this program is to protect the back (especially the lumbar region) as well as the neck and to strengthen the thighs.

🏋 **Do 2 or 3 circuits of 20 to 30 repetitions.**
▪ **Do this workout 1 or 2 times per week.**

❶ Straight-legged deadlift using continuous tension
▶ **P. 171**
❷ Crunch
▶ **P. 206**
❸ Leg extension using continuous tension
▶ **P. 166**
❹ Partial clean and jerk with continuous tension
▶ **P. 146**
❺ Twisting crunch
▶ **P. 207**
❻ Bent-over lateral raise
▶ **P. 104**
❼ Row
▶ **P. 134**
❽ Neck extension
▶ **P. 127**
❾ Neck flexion
▶ **P. 127**
❿ Lateral neck extension
▶ **P. 128**

Postworkout stretches
▶ **PP. 106/137/91**

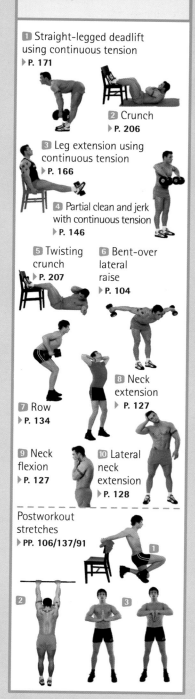

Phase 5: Customizing Your Program

After 12 to 18 months of weight training, you should personalize your training program to better meet the physical demands of your sport. Why should you wait so long to develop your program? Because it takes time to be able to tell what suits you best.

Your customized training program will be easy to plan so long as you understand exactly which muscles and which muscle qualities are required for your sport. You should also analyze your weaknesses so that you better understand how to improve them. And you must take into account the most common injury risks in your sport.

How to Analyze the Physical Requirements of Your Sport

To develop your training program, you need to do an individual analysis of your performance. This analysis has three main parts:

1. Which muscle groups are used?

With the programs in phase 4, you discovered the muscles that are most often used in the main athletic disciplines. Ideally, however, you should be able to feel on your own which muscles are most involved in your particular sport. Athletes who are most aware of their muscles at work make the quickest progress in weight training and on the playing field. Some people become aware of their muscle work early, while others never really feel it. This can lead the latter group to use hazardous and ineffective techniques to perform movements.

When you can feel your muscles perfectly, it is easier to make them work as they were designed to. This lets you learn a new movement faster and perform it more precisely. Weight training helps you develop this muscle sense, which will help improve your performance.

Once you are aware of your muscles, your muscular sensations will improve and you will have acquired a certain level of control over your body. It will also be easier for you to modify the workouts in phase 4 in order to develop your own weight training program.

2. What are the strengths and muscle qualities required for your sport?

In your sport, do you need pure strength, power, and speed, or a mixture of strength and endurance? It is rare to find a sport that uses only a single muscle quality. In general, sports involve a combination of several distinct qualities. However, there are a few muscle qualities that are often necessary in many sports, and we need to highlight those.

Pure strength. This happens when you need to move the heaviest object possible. To gain pure strength, you have to work with heavy weights and few repetitions. Pure strength is, however, rarely used by itself because, in general, a need for either speed or precision goes along with it.

Starting strength. This strength is used when you have to sprint as quickly as possible from a stationary position. Weight training with the stop-and-go technique helps to develop starting strength. For example, when doing a box squat, you stay seated for one or two seconds before exploding up using the strength of your thighs.

Acceleration strength. The goal is to accelerate when the body is already in motion. A typical example is escaping someone who is chasing you. You work on this quality in the opposite way that you work on starting strength. You combine the negative phase with the positive phase of a movement as rapidly as possible while maintaining continuous tension (do not fully straighten your arms or legs during weight training exercises).

Power and explosiveness. The object that needs to be moved (often, your own body) is not necessarily heavy. However, you need to move the object as quickly as possible. To work on power, you generally need to use a weight that is about 40 percent of your maximum so that the weight will not slow down your execution of the movement. The movement should be as fast as possible. To increase power, you should ideally combine resistance from dumbbells and resistance from bands. Plyometric training is also important.

Strength and endurance. Numerous sports require a combination of strength and endurance. To better associate these requirements, you must train in a nonstop circuit while doing several repetitions (at least 25 for the majority of the workout). Only a few sets should be done with heavy weights for approximately 12 repetitions. Continuous tension and tapering sets are two techniques that you should use often for increasing intensity.

3. What weaknesses keep you from progressing?

Among the muscle qualities used in your sport as well as the muscle groups involved in those movements, which are the least developed in your body? Which ones slow down your progress? Above all, your training program needs to focus on those qualities and those muscles. This seems obvious, but it often does not happen. Many athletes find it easier to work on their strong points than their weak ones.

Preventing Injury

All physical activities can lead to associated injuries. The slightest pain will diminish performance, interfere with training, and limit your development. Strengthening muscles at the site can prevent injury and enhance performance by consolidating these "weak links" in the muscle chain. We have included a few of these specific circuits in the workout programs in phase 4. This inclusion should be intensified when you develop your program.

Preventing Shoulder Pain

Sports that require a lot of shoulder movement can easily lead to deltoid pain. This happens in throwing sports (such as basketball, volleyball, handball, and shot put), combat sports, tennis, water sports, swimming, arm wrestling, climbing, and golf. To prevent pain, you must maintain stability in the joint and strengthen the support muscles (back of the shoulder, infraspinatus, and lower-trapezius muscles).

🕐 Do 3 to 5 circuits of 15 to 25 repetitions at least 2 times per week at the very beginning of your workout as a warm-up.

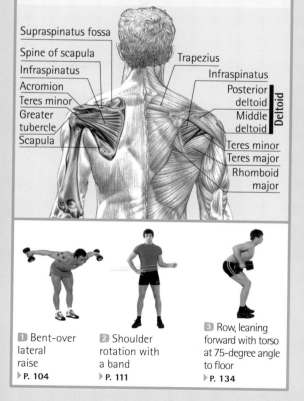

- Supraspinatus fossa
- Spine of scapula
- Infraspinatus
- Acromion
- Teres minor
- Greater tubercle
- Scapula
- Trapezius
- Infraspinatus
- Posterior deltoid
- Middle deltoid
- Deltoid
- Teres minor
- Teres major
- Rhomboid major

1 Bent-over lateral raise
▶ P. 104

2 Shoulder rotation with a band
▶ P. 111

3 Row, leaning forward with torso at 75-degree angle to floor
▶ P. 134

Preventing Lower-Back Pain

Almost all physical activities affect the spine, and the lower back is the most heavily worked. To prevent lower-back pain, you must strengthen the muscles that support the spine (the abdominal muscles, especially the lower muscles; the oblique muscles; and the latissimus dorsi muscles).

🕐 Do 2 to 4 circuits of 15 to 25 repetitions 2 or 3 times per week.
Do this circuit at the end of your workout.

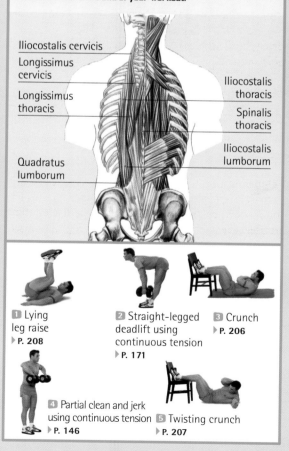

- Iliocostalis cervicis
- Longissimus cervicis
- Longissimus thoracis
- Quadratus lumborum
- Iliocostalis thoracis
- Spinalis thoracis
- Iliocostalis lumborum

1 Lying leg raise
▶ P. 208

2 Straight-legged deadlift using continuous tension
▶ P. 171

3 Crunch
▶ P. 206

4 Partial clean and jerk using continuous tension
▶ P. 146

5 Twisting crunch
▶ P. 207

Preventing Neck Pain

In contact sports (such as combat sports and rugby), the neck is heavily worked. To protect it, you must strengthen the muscles that maintain neck control as well as the upper-trapezius muscles.

⚡ **Do 2 to 4 circuits of the following:**
- **8 to 12 repetitions for shrugs and clean and jerk lifts**
- **20 to 30 repetitions for neck exercises**

Do this circuit at least 2 times per week at the end of your workout.

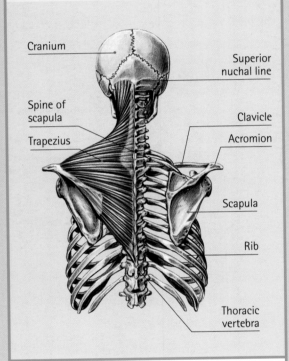

Cranium

Superior nuchal line

Spine of scapula

Trapezius

Clavicle

Acromion

Scapula

Rib

Thoracic vertebra

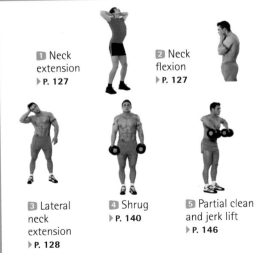

1 Neck extension
▶ **P. 127**

2 Neck flexion
▶ **P. 127**

3 Lateral neck extension
▶ **P. 128**

4 Shrug
▶ **P. 140**

5 Partial clean and jerk lift
▶ **P. 146**

Preventing Hip Pain

Sports that require hip rotation can easily damage the small muscles that control the movement of the thighs. This happens in ball sports, racket sports, combat sports, skiing, climbing, horseback riding, and ice sports.

⚡ **Do 2 or 3 circuits of 20 to 50 repetitions at least 2 times per week. Instead of directly combining the sets, take a 30-second break between sets and stretch the muscles you have just exercised. Include this circuit at the beginning of your workout as a warm-up.**

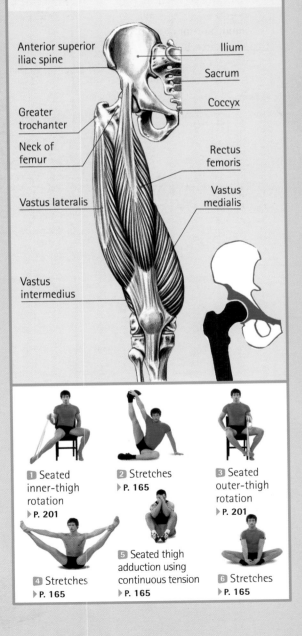

Anterior superior iliac spine

Ilium

Sacrum

Coccyx

Greater trochanter

Neck of femur

Rectus femoris

Vastus lateralis

Vastus medialis

Vastus intermedius

1 Seated inner-thigh rotation
▶ **P. 201**

2 Stretches
▶ **P. 165**

3 Seated outer-thigh rotation
▶ **P. 201**

4 Stretches
▶ **P. 165**

5 Seated thigh adduction using continuous tension
▶ **P. 165**

6 Stretches
▶ **P. 165**

Preventing Knee Pain

Knee problems are very common in sports. They occur most often in ball sports, racket sports, combat sports, running, skiing, biking, climbing, and rowing.

Knee problems happen so often because of a double imbalance:

1. Imbalance between the strength of the hamstrings and that of the quadriceps. Weight training programs generally focus on the quadriceps and neglect the hamstrings even though the hamstrings are much more important for movement.
2. Imbalance between the strength of the four muscles that make up the quadriceps. Naturally, these muscles do not pull on the kneecap with equal force.

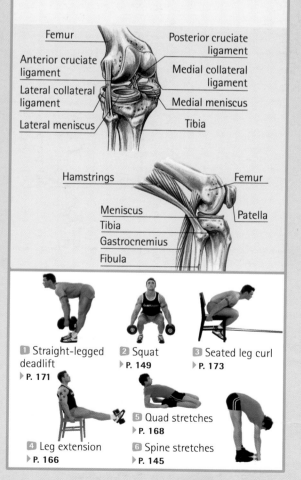

Femur

Anterior cruciate ligament

Lateral collateral ligament

Lateral meniscus

Posterior cruciate ligament

Medial collateral ligament

Medial meniscus

Tibia

Hamstrings

Meniscus

Tibia

Gastrocnemius

Fibula

Femur

Patella

1 Straight-legged deadlift
▶ **P. 171**

2 Squat
▶ **P. 149**

3 Seated leg curl
▶ **P. 173**

4 Leg extension
▶ **P. 166**

5 Quad stretches
▶ **P. 168**

6 Spine stretches
▶ **P. 145**

Preventing Hamstring Muscle Tears

Hamstring muscle tears are very common in running, particularly if it involves sprinting in an irregular fashion as in soccer, rugby, racket sports, ice skating, and track and field.

A four-year medical study on soccer players who were playing at a very high level shows that a regular stretching program alone has no impact on injuries. However, weight training with negative repetitions reduced the incidence of tears. The best results were obtained when negative repetitions and stretching were combined.

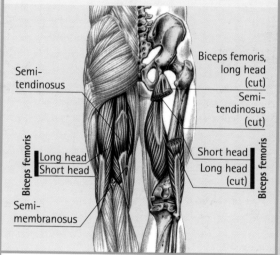

Semi-tendinosus

Biceps femoris

Semi-membranosus

Biceps femoris, long head (cut)

Semi-tendinosus (cut)

Long head
Short head

Short head

Long head (cut)

Biceps femoris

 1 Straight-legged deadlift:
Do the descending part of the exercise on the right leg only. Once your torso is parallel to the floor, put your left foot on the floor so that you can use both legs to raise your torso back up. Begin another negative repetition on the left leg while lifting your right foot off the floor.
Do 3 to 5 sets of 15 to 20 repetitions per leg (30 to 40 repetitions total).
Begin using a dumbbell in one hand once you are capable of doing 20 repetitions per leg.
▶ **P. 171**

 2 Seated leg curl:
Bring your feet under the chair using both your thighs. For the set on the right leg, your left foot will push on the right foot in order to bring the thigh into position. For the negative phase, hold the elastic band on the right foot only. Once the hamstring set is done, move on to the left thigh.
▶ **P. 173**
Do 3 or 4 sets of 10 to 15 repetitions per thigh.

255

Library of Congress Cataloging-in-Publication Data

Delavier, Frédéric.
  [Méthode Delavier de Musculation. English]
  The strength training anatomy workout / Frédéric Delavier, Michael Gundill.
      p. cm.
  Rev. ed. of: Méthode Delavier de Musculation. Paris : Éditions Vigot, 2009.
  ISBN-13: 978-1-4504-0095-4 (soft cover)
  ISBN-10: 1-4504-0095-7 (soft cover)
  1. Muscles--Anatomy. 2. Weight training. 3. Muscle strength. I. Gundill, Michael. II. Title.
  QM151.D45613 2011
  612.7'4--dc22
                              2010045127

ISBN-10: 1-4504-0095-7 (print)
ISBN-13: 978-1-4504-0095-4 (print)

Copyright © 2011 by Éditions Vigot, 23 rue de l'École de Médecine, 75006 Paris, France

This publication is written and published to provide accurate and authoritative information relevant to the subject matter presented. It is published and sold with the understanding that the author and publisher are not engaged in rendering legal, medical, or other professional services by reason of their authorship or publication of this work. If medical or other expert assistance is required, the services of a competent professional person should be sought.

This book is a revised edition of *La Méthode Delavier de Musculation,* published in 2009 by Éditions Vigot.

Illustrator: Frédéric Delavier

Human Kinetics books are available at special discounts for bulk purchase. Special editions or book excerpts can also be created to specification. For details, contact the Special Sales Manager at Human Kinetics.

Printed in France by Pollina - L57834A   10 9 8 7 6 5 4 3 2

Human Kinetics
Web site: www.HumanKinetics.com

United States: Human Kinetics
P.O. Box 5076
Champaign, IL 61825-5076
800-747-4457
e-mail: humank@hkusa.com

Canada: Human Kinetics
475 Devonshire Road Unit 100
Windsor, ON N8Y 2L5
800-465-7301 (in Canada only)
e-mail: info@hkcanada.com

Europe: Human Kinetics
107 Bradford Road
Stanningley
Leeds LS28 6AT, United Kingdom
+44 (0) 113 255 5665
e-mail: hk@hkeurope.com

Australia: Human Kinetics
57A Price Avenue
Lower Mitcham, South Australia 5062
08 8372 0999
e-mail: info@hkaustralia.com

New Zealand: Human Kinetics
P.O. Box 80
Torrens Park, South Australia 5062
0800 222 062
e-mail: info@hknewzealand.com

E5284